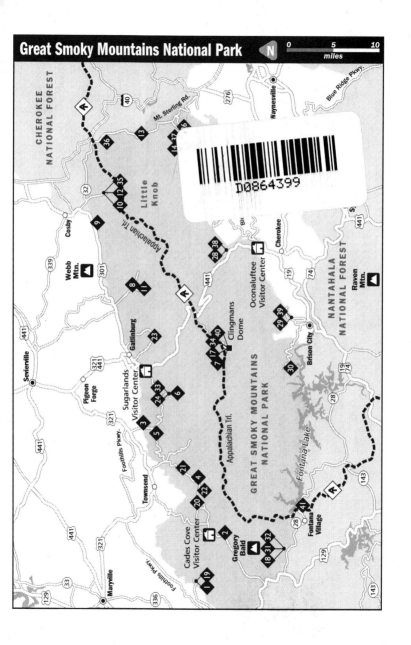

Map Key

Other Titles by the Author

Visit the author's Web site: www.johnnymolloy.com

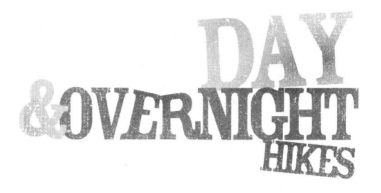

DAY
&OVERNIGHT
HIKES

Great Smoky Mountains National Park

Fourth Edition

JOHNNY MOLLOY

MENASHA RIDGE PRESS

DISCLAIMER

This book is meant only as a guide to select trails in the vicinity of Great Smoky Mountains National Park and does not guarantee hiker safety in any way—you hike at your own risk. Neither Menasha Ridge Press nor Johnny Molloy is liable for property loss or damage, personal injury, or death that result in any way from accessing or hiking the trails described in the following pages. Please be aware that hikers have been injured in the Great Smoky Mountains area. Be especially cautious when walking on or near boulders, steep inclines, and drop-offs, and do not attempt to explore terrain that may be beyond your abilities. To help ensure an uneventful hike, please read carefully the introduction to this book, and perhaps get further safety information and guidance from other sources. Familiarize yourself thoroughly with the areas you intend to visit before venturing out. Ask questions, and prepare for the unforeseen. Familiarize yourself with current weather reports, maps of the area you intend to visit, and any relevant park regulations.

Copyright © 2008 by Johnny Molloy
All rights reserved
Published by Menasha Ridge Press
Printed in the United States of America
Distributed by Publishers Group West
Fourth edition, first printing

Text and cover design by Ian Szymkowiak (Palace Press International)
Cartography and elevation profiles by Scott McGrew and Johnny Molloy

Library of Congress Cataloging-in-Publication Data

Molloy, Johnny, 1961–
    Day & overnight hikes, Great Smoky Mountains National Park /
        Johnny Molloy. — 4th ed.
        p. cm.
    Includes index.
    ISBN-13: 978-0-89732-662-9
    ISBN-10: 0-89732-662-8
    1. Hiking—Great Smoky Mountains National Park (N.C. and Tenn.)—
Guidebooks. 2. Backpacking—Great Smoky Mountains National Park (N.C.
and Tenn.)—Guidebooks. 3. Trails—Great Smoky Mountains National Park
(N.C. and Tenn.)—Guidebooks. 4. Great Smoky Mountains National Park
(N.C. and Tenn.)—Guidebooks. I. Title. II. Title: Day and overnight hikes,
Great Smoky Mountains National Park.
    GV199.42.G73M64 2008
    917.68'890454—dc22
                                    2008015799

Menasha Ridge Press
P.O. Box 43673
Birmingham, Alabama 35243
www.menasharidge.com

Table of Contents

PART I: GREAT OUT-AND-BACKS

TENNESSEE

Part II: Great Day Loops

Part III: Great Overnight Loops

Acknowledgments

Most books have only one person's name below the title—the author's. Thanks to Meredith Morris-Babb for steering me in the right direction, and to Mike Jones, Bud Zehmer, Nathan Lott, and the rest of the folks at Menasha Ridge Press. I would be remiss not to thank W. W. Armstrong, Jennifer Dyer, Nancy McBee, and my niece Jill Molloy for their help as well. Thanks to Aaron Marable for going on the latest Smokies hikes, too. Thanks to Bryan Delay, Karen Stokes, and John Cox for going backpacking in the Smokies over the years.

Dedication

This book is for Lisa Ann Daniel, who needs to take a hike.

Preface

Welcome to the fourth edition of this book. It has been a pleasure to keep this book up-to-date: It gives me more reasons to get back to the park where I cut my outdoor teeth. And what a park it is: 900 miles of trails, 500,000 acres of land, and some of the largest stands of old-growth forest in the East. The numbers of flora and fauna are just as impressive: 50 species of mammals, 80 species of fish, 200 species of birds, 1,300 species of flowering plants, 2,000 species of fungi, and more. The park boasts numerous trees of record dimensions among the upwards of 130 species that grow there. The diversity of ecosystems found in the Smokies is unmatched by that of any other temperate climate. Perhaps this is the reason for its impressive designation as both a national park and an international biosphere reserve.

To choose the Smokies as a place to spend your free time is a wise decision. And yet the Smokies can be intimidating, especially for the first-time visitor. Not only is there a lot of land to see, but with more than 9 million guests annually, the Great Smoky Mountains National Park is the most visited national park in the American system. Quite intimidating indeed. Thus, this book was conceived to make the real majesty of the Smokies accessible to visitors.

With so much land and so many people, discovering the beauty and solitude of this national park seems a hit-or-miss proposition. Where are the spectacular vistas? Where are the waterfalls and the old settlers' cabins? Where can I find solitude? Leaving it all to chance doesn't offer good odds for your all-too-brief vacation from the rat race. Weeks spent daydreaming of your fleeting slice of freedom could culminate in a three-hour driving marathon or a noisy walk up a crowded trail. Fortunately, with a little bit of planning and forethought, and this book, you can make the most of your time in the Smokies.

This book presents more than 30 day hikes for you to choose from. The majority of the hikes steer you toward infrequently visited areas, giving you the opportunity to enjoy your vacation on the trail instead of behind someone's car. These hikes offer solitude to maximize your Smoky Mountains experience, but, by necessity, portions of some hikes traverse popular and potentially crowded areas.

The day hikes offered here fall into one of two categories: out-and-back or loop. Out-and-back hikes take you to a particular rewarding destination and back on the same trail. The return trip allows you to see everything from the opposite vantage point. You may notice more minute features the second go-round, and retracing your steps at a different time of day can give the same trail a surprisingly different character.

To some, however, a return trip on the same trail isn't as enjoyable. Some hikers just can't stand the thought of covering the same ground twice, not with hundreds of untrodden Smokies miles awaiting them. Loop hikes avoid this. The loop hikes in this book are generally longer and harder than the out-and-back hikes, but a bigger challenge can reap bigger rewards.

Day hiking is the best and most popular way to "break into" the Smokies backcountry, but for those with the inclination, this book also offers ten overnight hikes. There are 102 designated backcountry sites and shelters available for those who want to capture the changing moods of the mountains. The length of these hikes, three days and two nights, accommodates those who have only an extended weekend. Longer trips are also available for those with more time. A permit is required for overnight stays in the backcountry. Certain campsites may be reserved in advance. Permits are available at visitor centers or by calling (865) 436-1231. Food storage cables have been installed at backcountry campsites. Please use them—you get to keep your food, and it keeps wild bears wild.

When visiting the Smokies, it's a great temptation to remain in your car, in part because auto tours, including one end of the famed Blue Ridge Parkway, abound. While auto touring is a great way to get an overview of the park, it creates a barrier between you and the mountains. Windshield tourists, hoping for a glimpse of bears and other wildlife, often end up seeing the tail end of the car in front of them. And while roadside overlooks offer easy views, the drone of traffic and lack of effort in reaching the views can make them less than inspirational. The Smokies were made for hiking.

The wilderness experience can unleash your mind and body, allowing you to relax and find peace and quiet. It also enables you to catch glimpses of beauty and splendor: a deer crashing through the underbrush as it clambers up a mountainside; the cabin remains of early settlers who scrabbled out a living among these woods; or a spectacular waterfall crashing above and below a trail. Out in these woods you can let your mind roam free, go where it pleases. This can't be achieved in a climate-controlled automobile.

The next few sections offer advice on how to use this book and how to have a safe and pleasant hike in the woods. The Smokies are a wild and beautiful place. I hope you will get out and enjoy what they have to offer.

—Johnny Molloy

Recommended Hikes

Introduction

How to Use This Guidebook

At the top of each hike profile is an information box that allows the hiker quick access to pertinent information: quality of scenery, difficulty of hike, condition of trail, expected degree of solitude, appropriateness for children, in addition to distance, approximate duration, and some highlights of the trip. The first five categories are rated using a five-star system. Below is an example of a box included with a hike:

31 Twentymile Loop

SCENERY: ✰ ✰ ✰ ✰ DIFFICULTY: ✰ ✰ TRAIL CONDITIONS: ✰ ✰ ✰ SOLITUDE: ✰ ✰ ✰ ✰ ✰ CHILDREN: ✰ ✰ ✰ ✰	DISTANCE: *7.4 miles round-trip* HIKING TIME: *3.75 hours round-trip* OUTSTANDING FEATURES: *Waterfall,* *mountain streams, deep woods*

On this hike, four stars indicate that the scenery will be picturesque, it will be a relatively easy climb (five stars for difficulty would be strenuous), the trail conditions are average (one star means the trail is likely to be muddy, narrow, or have some obstacle), you can expect to run into few if any people (with one star you'll likely be elbowing your way up the trail), and the hike is appropriate for able-bodied children (a one-star rating would denote that only the most gung-ho and physically fit children should go).

The distance is absolute, but the hiking time is an estimate for the average hiker making a round-trip. Overnight hiking times factor in the burden of carrying a pack and indicate the per-day hiking times.

Following each box is a brief description of the hike. A more detailed account follows, noting trail junctions, stream crossings, and trailside features, along with their distances from the trailhead. This helps keep you apprised of your whereabouts and makes sure you don't miss those features noted. You can use this guidebook to walk just a portion of a hike or to combine information to plan a hike of your own.

The hikes have been divided into out-and-back day hikes, loop day hikes, and overnight loops. The day hikes sections have been further divided into Tennessee and North Carolina hikes. Feel free to flip through the book, reading the descriptions and choosing a hike that appeals to you.

The Overview Map and Overview Map Key

Use the overview map on the inside front cover to assess the exact locations of each hike's primary trailhead. Each hike's number appears on the overview map, on the map key facing the overview map, and in the table of contents. Flipping through the book, you'll see a hike's full profile is easy to locate by watching for the hike number at the top of each page.

The book is organized by region as indicated in the table of contents. The hikes within each region are identified as one-way day hikes, loop day hikes, or overnight loop hikes. A map legend that details the symbols found on trail maps appears on the inside back cover.

Trail Maps

Each hike contains a detailed map that shows the trailhead, the route, significant features, facilities, and topographic landmarks such as creeks, overlooks, and peaks. The author gathered map data by carrying a GPS unit while hiking.

This data was downloaded into a digital mapping program and processed by expert cartographers to produce the highly accurate maps found in this book. Each trailhead's GPS coordinates are included with each profile.

ELEVATION PROFILES

Corresponding directly to the trail map, there is a detailed elevation profile for each hike. The elevation profile provides a quick look at the trail from the side, enabling you to visualize how the trail rises and falls. Key points along the way are labeled. Note the number of feet between each tick mark on the vertical axis (the height scale). To avoid making flat hikes look steep and steep hikes appear flat, height scales are used throughout the book to provide an accurate image of the hike's climbing difficulty.

GPS TRAILHEAD COORDINATES

The data was downloaded and plotted onto a digital USGS topo map. In addition to highly specific trail outlines, this book also includes the GPS coordinates for each trailhead in two formats: latitude/longitude and UTM. Latitude/longitude coordinates tell you where you are by locating a point west (latitude) of the 0° meridian line that passes through Greenwich, England, and north or south of the 0° (longitude) line that belts the Earth, aka the equator.

Topographic maps show latitude/longitude in addition to UTM grid lines. Known as UTM coordinates, the numbers index a specific point, using a grid method. The survey datum used to arrive at the coordinates in this book is WGS84 (versus NAD27 or WGS83). For readers who own a GPS unit, whether handheld or onboard a vehicle, the latitude/longitude or UTM coordinates provided on the first page of each hike may be entered into the GPS unit. Just make sure your GPS unit is set to navigate using WGS84 datum. Now you can navigate directly to the trailhead.

Most trailheads, which begin in parking areas, can be reached by car, but some hikes still require a short walk to reach the trailhead from a parking area. In those cases a handheld unit is necessary to continue the GPS navigation process. That said, readers can easily access all trailheads in this book by using the directions given, the overview map, and the trail map, which shows at least one major road leading into the area. But for those who enjoy using the latest GPS technology to navigate, the necessary data has been provided. A brief explanation of the UTM coordinates from Twentymile Loop follows.

Latitude	N35° 28' 9.9"
Longitude	W83° 52' 18.8"
UTM Zone	17S
Easting	0239350
Northing	3928700

The UTM zone number 17S refers to one of the 60 vertical zones of the Universal Transverse Mercator (UTM) projection. Each zone is 6 degrees wide. The easting number 0239350 indicates in meters how far east or west a point is from the central meridian of the zone. Increasing easting coordinates on a topo map or on your GPS screen indicate that you are moving east; decreasing easting coordinates indicate you are moving west. The northing number 3928700 references in meters how far you are from the equator. Above and below the equator, increasing northing coordinates indicate you are traveling north; decreasing northing coordinates indicate you are traveling south. To learn more about how to enhance your outdoor experiences with GPS technology, refer to *GPS Outdoors: A Practical Guide for Outdoor Enthusiasts* (Menasha Ridge Press).

Weather

The Smoky Mountains offer four distinct seasons for the hiker's enjoyment, but sometimes it seems all four are going on at once, depending on your location and elevation. Before your visit is over, you will probably see a little bit of everything. The chart below is from Gatlinburg, Tennessee, located just outside the park. Expect temperatures at higher elevations in the park to be 10°F –15°F cooler.

AVERAGE TEMPERATURE (F) BY MONTH IN GATLINBURG, TENNESSEE

	Jan	Feb	Mar	Apr	May	Jun
High	48°	52°	61°	69°	76°	82°
Low	25°	26°	33°	39°	49°	57°

	Jul	Aug	Sep	Oct	Nov	Dec
High	85°	84°	79°	70°	60°	51°
Low	62°	60°	54°	42°	33°	28°

Be prepared for a wide range of temperatures and conditions, no matter the season. As a rule of thumb, the temperature decreases about 3°F with every 1,000 feet of elevation gained. The Smokies are also the wettest place in the South. The park's higher elevations can receive upward of 90 inches of precipitation a year.

Spring, the most variable season, takes six weeks to reach the park's highest elevations. You may encounter both winter- and summerlike weather during April and May, often in the same day. As the weather warms, thunderstorms become more frequent. Summer days typically start clear, but as the day heats up, clouds build, often culminating in a heavy shower. Fall, the driest season, comes to the peaks in early September, working its way downhill, the reverse pattern of spring; warm days and cool nights are interspersed with less frequent wet periods.

Winter presents the Smokies at their most challenging. Frontal systems sweep through the region, with alternately cloudy and sunny days, though cloudy days are most frequent. No permanent snowpack exists in the high country, though elevations above 5,000 feet receive five feet of snow or more per year. The high country can see bitterly cold temperatures during this time. When venturing into the Smokies, it's a good idea to carry clothes for all weather extremes.

Water

How much is enough? Well, one simple physiological fact should convince you to err on the side of excess when deciding how much water to pack: A hiker working hard in 90°F heat needs approximately ten quarts of fluid per day. That's 2.5 gallons—12 large water bottles or 16 small ones. In other words, pack along 1 or 2 bottles, even for short hikes.

Some hikers and backpackers hit the trail prepared to purify water found along the route. This method, while less dangerous than drinking it untreated, comes with risks. Purifiers with ceramic filters are the safest. Many hikers pack along the slightly distasteful tetraglycine-hydroperiodide tablets to debug water (sold under the names Potable Aqua, Coughlan's, Aqua Mira, and others).

Probably the most common waterborne "bug" that hikers face is *Giardia lamblia,* which may not hit until one to four weeks after ingestion. It will have you living in the bathroom, passing noxious rotten-egg gas, vomiting, and shivering with chills. Other parasites to worry about include *E. coli* and *cryptosporidium,* both of which are harder to kill than *giardia.*

For most people, the pleasures of hiking make carrying water a relatively minor price to pay to remain healthy. If you're tempted to drink "found water," do so only if you understand the risks involved. Better yet, hydrate before your hike, carry (and drink) six ounces of water for every mile you plan to hike, and hydrate after the hike.

Clothing

There is a wide variety of clothing from which to choose. Basically, use common sense and be prepared for anything. If all you have are cotton clothes when a sudden rainstorm comes along, you'll be miserable, especially in cooler weather. It's a good idea to carry along a light wool sweater or some type of synthetic apparel (polypropylene, fleece, Thermax, etc.) and a hat.

Always carry raingear—preferably lined with Gore-Tex. Thunderstorms can come on suddenly in the summer, and winter fronts can soak you to the bone. Keep in mind that rainy days are as much a part of nature as are those idyllic days you desire. Besides, rainy days really cut down on the crowds. With appropriate raingear, you'll find a normally crowded trail can be a wonderful place of solitude. Do, however, remember that getting wet opens the door to hypothermia.

Footwear is another concern. Although tennis shoes may be appropriate for paved areas, many Smokies trails are rocky and rough; tennis shoes may not offer enough support. Waterproofed or not, boots should be your footwear of choice. Sport sandals are more popular than ever, but these leave much of your foot exposed. Injuring your foot when you are far from the trailhead can make for a miserable limp back to the car.

The Ten Essentials

One of the first rules of hiking is to be prepared for anything. The simplest way to be prepared is to carry the "ten essentials." In addition to carrying the items listed below, you need to know how to use them, especially the navigation items. Always consider worst-case scenarios, such as getting lost, hiking back in the dark, breaking gear (e.g., a broken hip strap on your pack or a plugged water filter), twisting an ankle, or encountering a brutal thunderstorm. The items listed below don't cost a lot of money, don't take up much room in a pack, and don't weigh much, but they might just save your life.

WATER: durable bottles, and water treatment such as iodine or a filter

MAP: preferably a topo map and a trail map with a route description

COMPASS: a high-quality compass

FIRST-AID KIT: a good-quality kit including first-aid instructions

KNIFE: a multitool device with pliers is best

LIGHT: flashlight or headlamp with extra bulbs and batteries

FIRE: windproof matches or lighter and fire starter

EXTRA FOOD: you should always have food in your pack when you've finished hiking

EXTRA CLOTHES: rain protection, warm layers, gloves, warm hat

SUN PROTECTION: sunglasses, lip balm, sunblock, sun hat

First-Aid Kit

A typical first-aid kit may contain more items than you might think necessary. These are just the basics. Prepackaged kits in waterproof bags (Atwater Carey and Adventure Medical make a variety of kits) are available. Even though there are quite a few items listed here, they pack down into a small space:

Ace bandages or Spenco joint wraps

Antibiotic ointment (Neosporin or the generic equivalent)

Aspirin or acetaminophen

Band-Aids

Benadryl or the generic equivalent diphenhydramine (in case of allergic reactions)

Butterfly-closure bandages

Epinephrine in a prefilled syringe (for people known to have severe allergic reactions to such things as bee stings)

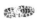

Gauze (one roll)

Gauze compress pads (a half dozen 4 x 4-inch pads)

Hydrogen peroxide or iodine

Insect repellent

Matches or pocket lighter

Moleskin/Spenco 2nd Skin

Sunscreen

Whistle (it's more effective in signaling rescuers than your voice is)

Hiking with Children

No one is too young for a hike in the outdoors. Be mindful, though. Flat, short, and shaded trails are best with an infant. Toddlers who have not quite mastered walking can still tag along, riding on an adult's back in a child carrier. Use common sense to judge a child's capacity to hike a particular trail, and always anticipate that the child will tire quickly and need to be carried. A list of hikes suitable for children is provided on page xii.

General Safety

To some potential mountain enthusiasts, the deep woods seem inordinately dark, perilous, and full of hazards. It is the fear of the unknown that causes this anxiety. No doubt, potentially dangerous situations can occur in the outdoors, but as long as you use sound judgment and prepare yourself before you hit the trail, you'll be much safer in the woods than in most urban areas in our country. It is better to look at a backcountry hike as a fascinating discovery of the unknown, rather than a potential for disaster. Here are a few tips to make your trip safer and easier:

- **ALWAYS BRING FOOD AND WATER, EVEN WHEN DAY HIKING.**
Food will give you energy, help keep you warm, and in an emergency situation may sustain you until help arrives. And you never know if you will find a stream nearby when you are thirsty. Of course, if you drink water from a stream, purify it first. The chance of getting sick from *giardia* or other waterborne organisms is small, but there is no reason to take a chance. Boil, filter, or treat all water before drinking it. Outdoor retailers offer a wide range of water filters and purification tablets.

- **STAY ON DESIGNATED TRAILS.** Most hikers get lost when they leave the trail. If you become disoriented, don't panic—this may result in a bad decision that will make your predicament worse. Retrace your steps if you can remember them, or stay put. Rangers check the trails first when searching for lost or overdue hikers.

- **BRING A MAP, COMPASS, AND LIGHTER,** and know how to use a map and compass. Should you become lost, these three items can help you stick around long enough to be found or get yourself out of a pickle. Trail maps are available at visitor centers and ranger stations. A compass can help you orient yourself, and a lighter can start a fire (for heat or for signaling). A GPS can help you locate your position.

- **BE ESPECIALLY CAREFUL CROSSING STREAMS.** Whether you are fording the stream or crossing it on a footlog, make every step count. If using a footlog, hold on to the handrail, and be aware that footlogs are often moss covered and slippery. When fording a stream, use a trekking pole or stout limb as a third leg for balance. If a stream seems too high to ford, turn back.

- **BE AWARE OF THE SYMPTOMS OF HYPOTHERMIA.** Shivering and forgetfulness are the two most prevalent indicators of this cold-weather killer, which can occur even in the summer (at higher elevations), especially when a hiker is wearing wet clothing. If symptoms arise, find the victim warm shelter, hot liquids, and dry clothes or a sleeping bag.

- **AVOID BEAR-FEAR PARALYSIS.** The black bears of the Smokies are wild animals and hence unpredictable. If you see one, give it a wide berth; don't feed it and you'll be fine. Most injuries have occurred when an ignorant visitor fed or otherwise harassed a wild bear.

· **ALWAYS BRING RAINGEAR.** The Smokies are the wettest place in the East, which is an important factor in their remarkable biodiversity. Keep in mind that a rainy day is as much a part of nature as are those idyllic sunny days; and rainy days tend to keep the crowds at bay. With the appropriate raingear, a normally crowded trail can afford solitude. Do remember that getting wet opens the door to hypothermia.

· **TAKE ALONG YOUR BRAIN.** A cool, calculating mind is the single most important piece of equipment you'll ever need on the trail. Think before you act. Watch your step. Plan ahead. Avoiding accidents before they happen is the best plan for a rewarding, stress-relieving hike.

· **ASK QUESTIONS.** Park employees are there to help. It's a lot easier to seek advice beforehand than to have a mishap away from civilization. Use your head out there, and treat the place as if it were your own backyard. After all, it is your national park.

Animal and Plant Hazards

TICKS

Ticks like to hang out in the brush that grows along trails, especially on dry ridges. Hot summer months seem to explode their numbers. Ticks, which are arthropods and not insects, need a host to feast on in order to reproduce. The ticks that light onto you while hiking will be very small, sometimes so tiny that you won't be able to spot them. Primarily of two varieties, deer ticks and dog ticks, both need a few hours of actual attachment before they can transmit any disease they may harbor. Ticks may settle in shoes, socks, hats, and may take several hours to actually latch on. The best strategy is to visually check every half-hour or so while hiking, do a thorough check before you get in the car, and then, when you take a posthike shower, do an even more thorough check of your entire body. Ticks that haven't attached are easily removed, but not easily killed. If you pick off a tick in the woods, just toss it aside. If you find one on your body at home, dispatch it and then send it down the toilet. For ticks that have embedded, removal with tweezers is best.

SNAKES

Spend some time hiking the Smokies and you may be surprised by the area's variety of snakes—18 in all. Most encounters will be with nonvenomous specimens. Only two poisonous snakes call the

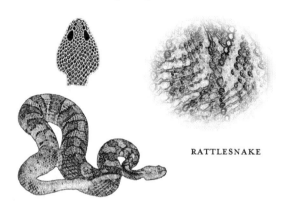

RATTLESNAKE

park home: the copperhead and the timber rattler. Copperheads can be found near streams and on outcrops, whereas rattlers will primarily be seen sunning on rocks. Spend a few minutes studying snakes before heading into the woods; a good rule of thumb is to give whatever animal you encounter a wide berth and leave it alone.

POISON IVY/POISON OAK/POISON SUMAC

Recognizing poison ivy, oak, and sumac and avoiding contact with them is the most effective way to prevent the painful, itchy rashes associated with these plants. In the Southeast, poison ivy ranges from a thick, tree-hugging vine to a shaded groundcover, three leaflets to a leaf; poison oak occurs as either a vine or shrub, with three leaflets as well; and poison sumac flourishes in swampland, each leaf

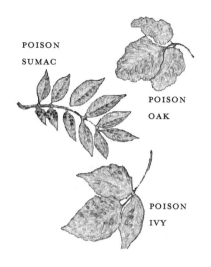

POISON
SUMAC

POISON
OAK

POISON
IVY

containing 7 to 13 leaflets. Urushiol, the oil in the sap of these plants, is responsible for the rash. Usually within 12 to 14 hours of exposure (but sometimes much later), raised lines and/or blisters will appear, accompanied by a terrible itch. Refrain from scratching; bacteria under fingernails can cause infection, and you will spread the rash to other parts of your body. Wash and dry the rash thoroughly, applying a calamine lotion or other product to help dry the rash. If the itching or blistering is severe, seek medical attention. Remember that oil-contaminated clothes, pets, or hiking gear can easily cause an irritating rash on you or someone else, so wash not only any exposed parts of your body but also clothes, gear, and pets.

Tips for Enjoying Smoky Mountains National Park

Before you go, call the national park for an information kit at (865) 436-1200. This will help get you oriented to the roads, features, and attractions of the Smokies. Another helpful source of information is the Great Smoky Mountains National Park Web site: **www.nps.gov/grsm.**

The following tips will make your visit enjoyable and more rewarding:

· GET OUT OF YOUR CAR AND ONTO A TRAIL. Auto touring merely allows a cursory overview of the park, mostly from a visual perspective. On the trail there are more scents and sounds. This guidebook recommends some trails over others, but any trail is better than no trail.

· USE OUTLYING TRAILHEADS TO START A HIKE. First, you will avoid the traffic on the main roads. Second, you're more likely to encounter solitude on the outlying trails than on trails off the main roads. The park is big, yet most visitors congregate in a few areas, so branch out.

· INVESTIGATE DIFFERENT AREAS OF THE PARK. The Smokies offer a wide variety of elevation, terrain, and forest types. You'll be pleasantly surprised to see so many distinct landscapes in one national park. Detailed USGS maps are on sale at the visitor centers.

· TAKE YOUR TIME ALONG THE TRAILS. Pace yourself. The Smokies are filled with wonders both big and small. Don't rush past a unique salamander to get to that overlook. Stop and smell the wildflowers. Listen to the woods around you. Peer into the clear mountain stream. Don't miss the trees for the forest.

· WE CAN'T ALWAYS SCHEDULE OUR FREE TIME WHEN WE WANT, but try to hike during the week and avoid the traditional holidays if possible. Trails that are packed in the summer are often clear during the colder seasons. If you are hiking on busy days, go early in the morning; it'll enhance your chances of seeing wildlife, too. The trails really clear out during rainy times. However, don't hike during a thunderstorm.

Backcountry Advice

Be sure to get the required (but free) backcountry-camping permit before you embark on your overnight trip. You can get a permit in person at entrance stations, visitor centers, park headquarters, and some self-registration stations. Plan your trip before obtaining your permit. Backcountry camping is allowed only at designated backcountry campsites. Solid human waste must be buried in a hole

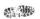

at least three inches deep and at least 20 yards from trails and water sources; a trowel is basic backpacking equipment. Otherwise, "pack it in, pack it out." Practice "leave no trace" camping ethics while in the backcountry. You are required to hang your food out of reach of bears and other animals in order to minimize the human impact on wildlife and to avoid these animals' introduction to and dependence on human food. Wildlife learns to associate backpacks and backpackers with easy food sources, thereby influencing their behavior. Foot storage cables have been installed at every backcountry campsite to facilitate food hanging.

It may seem a backcountry trip is fraught with rules and regulations, but the whole scheme is designed to foster a pleasant, safe, low-impact interaction between people and the rest of nature. The rules are intended to enhance your experience within the confines of this Southern Appalachian refuge. Note that park regulations can change over time; contact the park to confirm the status of the above regulations before you enter the backcountry.

Trail Etiquette

Whether you're on a city, county, state, or national park trail, always remember that great care and resources (from both nature and your tax dollars) have gone into creating these trails. Treat the trail, wildlife, and fellow hikers with respect.

· HIKE ON OPEN TRAILS ONLY. Respect trail and road closures (ask if you're not sure), avoid trespassing on private land, and obtain all required permits and authorization. Also, leave gates as you found them or as marked.

· LEAVE ONLY FOOTPRINTS. Be sensitive to the ground beneath you. This also means staying on the existing trail and not blazing any new trails. Be sure to pack out what you pack in. No one likes to see the trash someone else has left behind.

- **NEVER SPOOK ANIMALS.** An unannounced approach, a sudden movement, or a loud noise startles most animals. A surprised animal can be dangerous to you, to others, and to themselves. Give them plenty of space.

- **PLAN AHEAD.** Know your equipment, your ability, and the area in which you are hiking—and prepare accordingly. Be self-sufficient at all times; carry necessary supplies for changes in weather or other conditions. A well-executed trip is a satisfaction to you and to others.

- **BE COURTEOUS TO YOUR FELLOW HIKERS,** bikers, equestrians, and others you encounter on the trails.

IMPORTANT SMOKIES PHONE NUMBERS

Park Headquarters: (865) 436-1200
Park Natural History Association: (865) 436-0120
Developed Camping Reservations: (800) 365-2267
Backcountry Information: (865) 436-1297
Backcountry Camping Reservations: (865) 436-1231

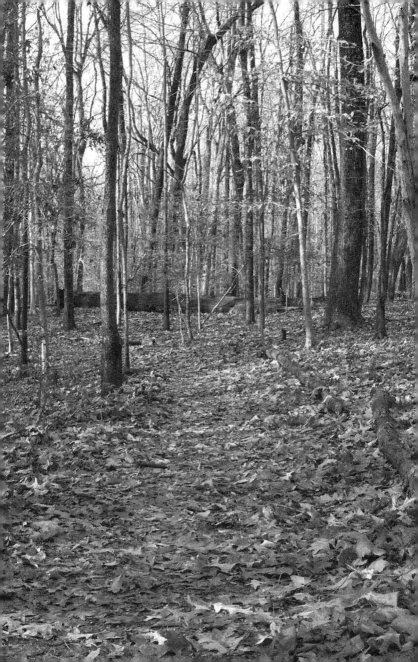

part one
GREAT OUT AND BACKS

1

The return
trip to the
AT will
get you
huffing and
puffing
while
thinking of
all the
people that
skipped
this
second view
as is
evidenced
by the
much less
used trail
tread

SCENERY: ☆ ☆ ☆ ☆ ☆	DISTANCE: *9.8 miles round-trip*
DIFFICULTY: ☆ ☆	HIKING TIME: *5.5 hours round-trip*
TRAIL CONDITIONS: ☆ ☆ ☆	OUTSTANDING FEATURES: *Abrams Creek*
SOLITUDE: ☆ ☆ ☆	*gorge, Abrams Falls*
CHILDREN: ☆ ☆ ☆	

It's hard to believe how few people you'll see taking this route to the popular Abrams Falls. The sounds of Abrams Creek will keep you company for most of the hike, though. This hike starts on Cooper Road Trail, behind the Abrams Creek campground. Follow this jeep road through a fading hemlock forest and across Kingfisher Creek, which can be a wet crossing in high water.

🏃🏃 At mile 0.9, turn right onto Little Bottoms Trail, which is hardly more than a glorified manway, as opposed to the wide jeep road that is Cooper Road Trail.

Begin a short but steep climb. After topping a small ridge, descend a short distance beyond the ridgetop. In a clearing on your right, between two of the area's many pine trees, you will find a spectacular view. On the trail's right, Abrams Creek gorge lines up with the Smokies crest as a backdrop, allowing a view from creek bottom to mountaintop. Continue winding down until you come to the creek. Cross several small branches along Abrams Creek, reaching Little Bottoms Backcountry Campsite 17, at mile 2.5.

Watch your step on this spare trail as it once again climbs the steep side of the gorge filled with the rumblings of Abrams Creek below. Winding in and out of small side hollows, it intersects the Hatcher Mountain Trail at mile 3.1. Keep forward, descending briefly, to intersect the Abrams Falls Trail at mile 3.3.

To the right, the Hannah Mountain Trail begins with a difficult ford of Abrams Creek. As you continue forward along

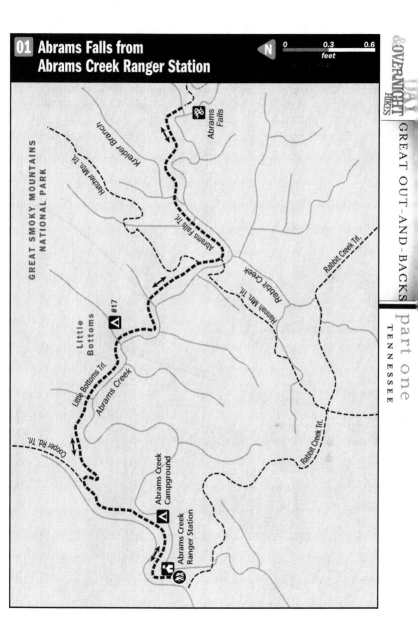

01 Abrams Falls from Abrams Creek Ranger Station

N

0   0.3   0.6
feet

&OVERNIGHT HIKES
DAY

GREAT SMOKY MOUNTAINS
NATIONAL PARK

Kreider Branch

Hatcher Mtn. Trl.

Abrams Falls

Abrams Falls Trl.

Rabbit Creek

Rabbit Creek Trl.

Hannah Mtn. Trl.

#17

Little
Bottoms

Little Bottoms Trl.

Abrams Creek

Cooper Rd. Trl.

Rabbit Creek Trl.

Abrams Creek
Campground

Abrams Creek
Ranger Station

Abrams Falls Trail—alternately crossing small creeks and looping around rib ridges on a footpath wider than the Little Bottoms Trail—Abrams Creek is always within earshot. At mile 4.9, arrive at the falls. You will be surprised to see crowds who have come 2.5 miles from Cades Cove. Enjoy the falls and the immense plunge pool before returning to the Abrams Creek Ranger Station.

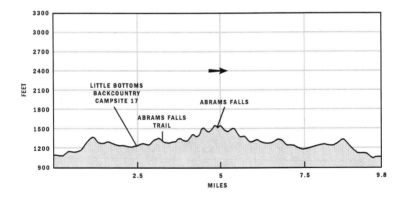

DIRECTIONS: From Townsend, Tennessee, drive west on US 321 and turn left onto Foothills Parkway. Follow Foothills Parkway west to US 129, and turn left onto US 129 at Chilhowee Lake. Head south 0.5 miles to Happy Valley Road. Turn left on Happy Valley Road, following it 6 miles to Abrams Creek Road. Turn right on Abrams Creek Road and drive 1 mile to the campground, passing the ranger station. Cooper Road Trail starts behind the campground. Park your car in the designated area near the ranger station.

GPS Trailhead Coordinates	01 ABRAMS FALLS FROM ABRAMS CREEK RANGER STATION
Latitude:	N35° 36' 35.4"
Longitude:	W83° 56' 8.6"
UTM Zone (WGS 84):	17S
Easting:	0234072
Northing:	3944436

SCENERY: ☆ ☆ ☆ ☆ ☆	DISTANCE: *10.8 miles round-trip*
DIFFICULTY: ☆ ☆ ☆	HIKING TIME: *5.75 hours round-trip*
TRAIL CONDITIONS: ☆ ☆ ☆ ☆	OUTSTANDING FEATURES: *Gregory Bald,*
SOLITUDE: ☆ ☆ ☆	*views from grassy field, virgin forest*
CHILDREN: ☆ ☆ ☆	

This hike is packed with features to satisfy even the most demanding hiker. On the way to Gregory Bald, world renowned for its wildflowers, pass along a mountain stream surrounded by old growth woodland and ascend a ridge, then pass historic Moore Spring, where an Appalachian Trail shelter once stood. It's a steady climb to the bald but well worth it.

🚶🚶 Ascend quickly upon leaving Forge Creek Road to join up with Forge Creek proper, crossing it on a footbridge. A little more than a mile into the hike, an old-growth forest of tulip trees begins to dominate the mountain scenery. Tulip trees, formerly known as tulip poplars or just poplars, have been renamed, since they are not true poplars. Footlogs help you cross Forge Creek at miles 1.7 and 1.9. Just beyond the last crossing is Forge Creek Backcountry Campsite 12. Fill up with water here—the rest of the way is dry until Moore Spring.

Leave the valley behind for the drier slope of Gregory Ridge. Top out on the ridge at mile 3. You've worked hard to get here, but the ridge keeps on rising. Views of the Smokies to your left keep your spirits up as you near Rich Gap and a trail junction, which lies at mile 4.9.

Here, you will turn right on Gregory Bald Trail for the final 0.5-mile ascent to Gregory Bald. But first, follow the unmarked path straight ahead. To the left 0.1 mile on, Long Hungry Ridge Trail from Twentymile Ranger Station terminates. Continue straight another 0.2 miles to reach Moore Spring, where an Appalachian

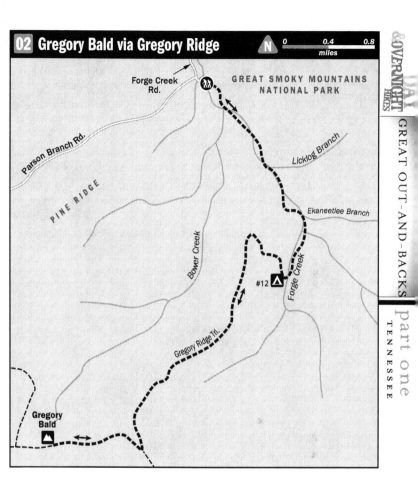

Forge Creek Rd.

GREAT SMOKY MOUNTAINS NATIONAL PARK

Parson Branch Rd.

PINE RIDGE

Licklog Branch

Ekaneetlee Branch

Bower Creek

Forge Creek

#12

Gregory Ridge Trl.

Gregory Bald

Trail (A.T.) shelter once stood before the A.T. was rerouted over Fontana Dam in the 1940s. The spring, in a small clearing that beckons you to stop, is one of the Smokies' finest. Remember to treat all water before drinking.

Return to Rich Gap and the trail junction. Turn left on Gregory Bald Trail, and soon you'll be on the bald, at mile 5.4. Earlier in this century, cattle grazing kept the forest from overtaking this hilltop clearing, or bald, and maintained a 15-acre open space. By the mid-1980s, the clearing had shrunk to less than half that size. The park service decided to return Gregory Bald to its original size. Nowadays, don't be surprised if you see the park service actually mowing and cutting back growth at the bald's edges. However, many of the flame azalea bushes are left intact to bloom profusely during June. A hungry hiker can also sample blueberries later in the summer. Except in inclement weather, Gregory Bald offers nearly 360-degree views year-round. Just a mile west is Parson Bald. To the south are the mountains of the Nantahala National Forest. Cades Cove lies below to the north, with East Tennessee and the Cumberland Mountains beyond.

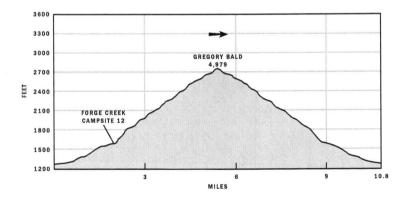

DIRECTIONS: Follow Cades Cove Loop Road 5.5 miles, then turn right on Forge Creek Road. Follow it 2.3 miles to the turnaround and the Gregory Ridge trailhead.

GPS Trailhead Coordinates	02 GREGORY BALD VIA
	GREGORY RIDGE
Latitude:	N35° 33' 45.5"
Longitude:	W83° 50' 46.1"
UTM Zone (WGS 84):	17S
Easting:	0242030
Northing:	3938950

03 Walker Sisters Place *via Little Greenbrier Trail*

SCENERY: ☆ ☆ ☆ ☆ ☆	DISTANCE: *5 miles round-trip*
DIFFICULTY: ☆ ☆	HIKING TIME: *2.75 hours*
TRAIL CONDITIONS: ☆ ☆ ☆ ☆	OUTSTANDING FEATURES: *Views, pioneer*
SOLITUDE: ☆ ☆ ☆ ☆	*homestead*
CHILDREN: ☆ ☆ ☆ ☆	

This scenic hike along a ridgeline offers views down to one of the last working pioneer homesteads in the Smokies. Start at a gap on Little Greenbrier Trail along the national park boundary. The views are numerous from a pine-cloaked mountainside before the second gap. Dip down to a hollow and reach Walker Sisters Place, which was occupied by spinster siblings until 1964.

🏃 Begin this hike at Wear Cove Gap on Little Greenbrier Trail. Climb through a classic pine-oak forest on a narrow pathway. This path skirts the park border in several places—you will see boundary signs here and there. Also, look down at the elaborate stonework by trail makers that keeps the path from tilting sideways with the mountainside.

Level out in a gap at 0.8 miles, then begin to swing around the south side of Little Mountain. There are good views into the heart of the park. Numerous dead pine snags are the result of the natural relationship between pines and the native pine beetle. There are also views into Wear Cove to the north and Cove Mountain to the east. Drop down the ridge of Little Mountain to reach Little Brier Gap and a trail junction at mile 1.9. Turn right here, on Little Brier Gap Trail, descending into the moist cove of Little Brier Branch, which lies to your left. Tulip trees join the forest. Pass a flat and a former clearing on the left.

Reach a gravel road at 2.3 miles and turn left, along tiny Straight Cove Branch. Come to an open area at 2.5 miles and reach

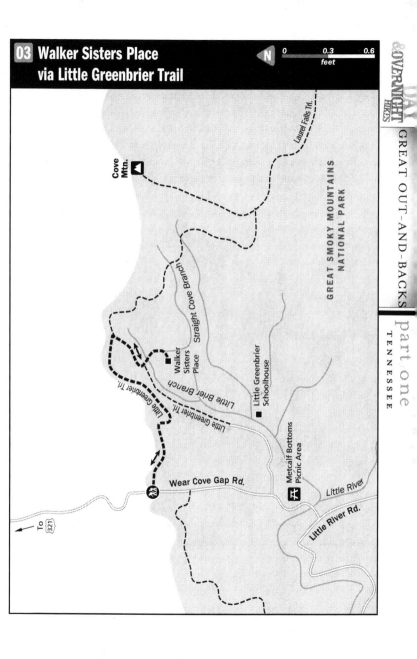

03 **Walker Sisters Place via Little Greenbrier Trail**

N

0   0.3   0.6
feet

Laurel Falls Trl.

Cove Mtn.

GREAT SMOKY MOUNTAINS NATIONAL PARK

Straight Cove Branch

Walker Sisters Place

Little Greenbrier Trl.

Little Brier Branch

Little Greenbrier Schoolhouse

Little Greenbrier Trl.

Metcalf Bottoms Picnic Area

Wear Cove Gap Rd.

To 321

Little River

Little River Rd.

Walker Sisters Place, in a grassy clearing. This cove was occupied for 150 years, with the Walker sisters remaining after the national park was established, thanks to a lifetime-lease agreement. After they passed away, the park preserved their homestead. Now, the springhouse, main home, and small barn remain. Notice the notched-log construction of the buildings and the nonnative ornamental bushes. If you are further interested in the area's history, continue down Little Brier Gap Trail 1.1 more miles to the Little Greenbrier Schoolhouse before returning to Wear Cove Gap.

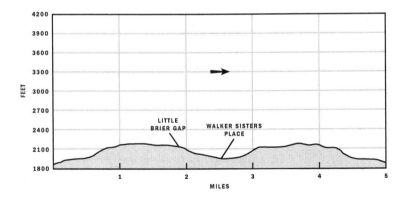

DIRECTIONS: From the park entrance at Townsend, drive straight to reach the Townsend "Wye." Turn left here, onto Little River Road, and follow it 7.8 miles to Metcalf Bottoms Picnic Area. Turn left into Metcalf Bottoms Picnic Area, crossing the Little River on a bridge. Continue on the road 1.3 miles to the park border, where Little Greenbrier Trail starts on the right. There is parking here for only one car, directly by the trail; another parking area is just over the hill from the trailhead.

GPS Trailhead Coordinates	03 WALKER SISTERS PLACE VIA LITTLE GREENBRIER TRAIL
Latitude:	N35° 41' 37.0"
Longitude:	W83° 38' 45.4"
UTM Zone (WGS 84):	17S
Easting:	0260571
Northing:	3953007

04 Rocky Top *via Lead Cove*

SCENERY: ☆ ☆ ☆ ☆ ☆
DIFFICULTY: ☆ ☆ ☆ ☆
TRAIL CONDITIONS: ☆ ☆ ☆ ☆
SOLITUDE: ☆ ☆ ☆ ☆
CHILDREN: ☆ ☆

DISTANCE: *11.4 miles round-trip*
HIKING TIME: *6 hours round-trip*
OUTSTANDING FEATURES: *Spence Field, 360-degree view from Rocky Top*

This hike is the epitome of the old adage, "You reap what you sow." You will burn a lot of calories on the climb to your destination, but the view is as good as views get. Leave the lowlands via Lead Cove Trail to intersect Bote Mountain Trail up to the Appalachian Trail, pass through Spence Field, and climb farther still to the storied Rocky Top.

🏃 Leave Laurel Creek Road behind and step into history on Lead Cove Trail, for what is a hike in the Smokies without a little history? Lead Cove derived its name from the ore that was extracted here in the 1800s. Soon you pass an old homesite that lingers among the cool forest of the cove. Keep climbing somewhat steeply, leaving the bottomland behind to arrive at Sandy Gap and Bote Mountain Trail at mile 1.8.

Turn right on the ridge-running jeep trail to Bote Mountain. Ascend steadily through the fairly open pine-oak forest that allows intermittent views of Defeat Ridge to your left. At mile 3, you'll pass through Anthony Creek Trail junction then come to a jeep turnaround at mile 3.7. The trail becomes furrowed and narrow, passing through a seemingly continuous rhododendron tunnel to arrive at a saddle on Spence Field at mile 4.7.

Turn left on the famed Appalachian Trail, skirting Spence Field's eastern flank. Continue alongside the grassy meadow, passing Jenkins Ridge Trail at mile 5.1. You'll descend briefly only to begin the final 0.6-mile climb to Rocky Top (elevation 5,441 feet) and

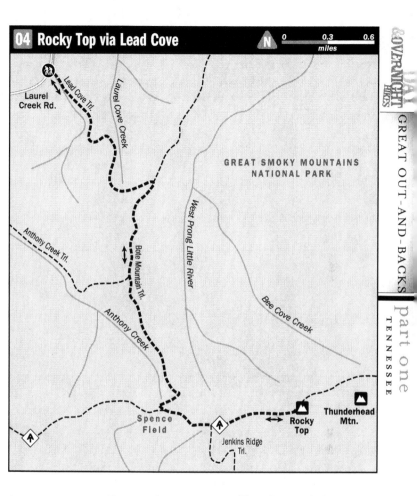

N

0   0.3   0.6
miles

Laurel
Creek Rd.

Lead Cove Trl.

Laurel Cove Creek

GREAT SMOKY MOUNTAINS
NATIONAL PARK

Anthony Creek Trl.

Bote Mountain Trl.

West Prong Little River

Anthony Creek

Bee Cove Creek

Spence
Field

Jenkins Ridge
Trl.

Rocky
Top

Thunderhead
Mtn.

its awesome views. Once at the summit, you'll understand why the
view inspired the famed country song *Rocky Top*. The tune doubles
as fight song for the University of Tennessee, which lies a mere
30 miles to the northwest. To your west, the meadows of Spence

Field and the western crest of the Smokies, all the way to Shuckstack Mountain, stand out in bold relief. The views into Tennessee and North Carolina extend to the horizon. To your east, the prominent peak with the imposing name of Thunderhead competes with the sky. Take in the view from this rock outcrop just as others have done for generations.

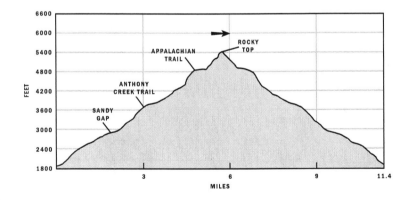

DIRECTIONS: From the park entrance at Townsend, Tennessee, head forward to the Townsend "Wye." Turn right here onto Laurel Creek Road and follow it 5.6 miles southwest towards Cades Cove. Lead Cove Trail is on your left, just beyond a small parking area that extends on both sides of the road.

GPS Trailhead Coordinates	04 ROCKY TOP VIA LEAD COVE
Latitude:	N35° 36' 18.6"
Longitude:	W83° 44' 40.8"
UTM Zone (WGS 84):	17S
Easting:	0251360
Northing:	3943410

05 Buckhorn Gap *via Meigs Creek*

SCENERY: ✪ ✪ ✪ ✪	DISTANCE: *6.8 miles round-trip*
DIFFICULTY: ✪ ✪	HIKING TIME: *3 hours round-trip*
TRAIL CONDITIONS: ✪ ✪ ✪	OUTSTANDING FEATURES: *Meigs Creek Valley*
SOLITUDE: ✪ ✪ ✪ ✪ ✪	
CHILDREN: ✪ ✪ ✪	

Once you leave the crowds at The Sinks behind, you'll probably have this intimate slice of the Smokies to yourself. This trail allows you to notice the smaller subtle features of a Southern Appalachian mountain valley. Meigs Creek will surely catch your eye; you cross it nearly 20 times. Not to worry, though: most crossings are not difficult in times of normal water flow. However, stay off this trail if the water is up.

🚶 Once on Meigs Creek Trail, swing past The Sinks, a popular swimming and sunbathing spot. Immediately drop into a boggy area, unusual for the Smokies, that was once part of the Little River. Begin ascending onto a dry, piney ridge and notice the change in forest from the Little River Valley. Wind back down and finally encounter the trail's namesake, Meigs Creek, at mile 1.

The crossings begin here as the creek and trail merge amid a dark-green forest interspersed with crashing cascades that flow beneath thickets of rhododendron. After the fourth crossing, a particularly comely falls announces its presence on your right. Continue fording, but stop to notice the clarity of the stream. The people who settled these coves revered their Smoky Mountain water and couldn't get used to drinking "still" well water after they left their highland homes.

As you continue to climb slightly, Meigs Creek and the side creeks that feed it become smaller. Toward the head of the valley, you'll notice that loggers left certain large hemlock trees, now succumbing to hemlock woolly adelgid, behind. They were not

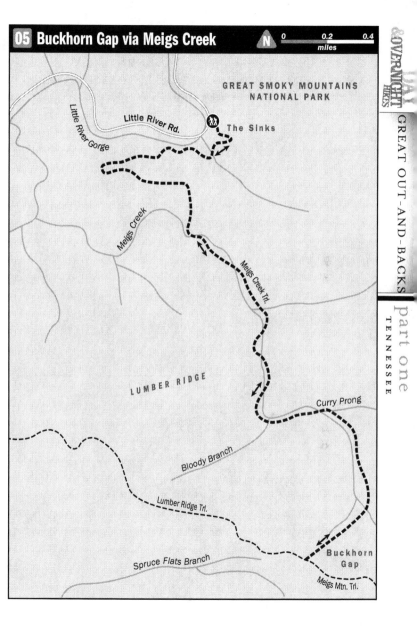

N

0   0.2   0.4
miles

GREAT SMOKY MOUNTAINS
NATIONAL PARK

Little River Rd.

The Sinks

Little River Gorge

Meigs Creek

Meigs Creek Trl.

LUMBER RIDGE

Curry Prong

Bloody Branch

Lumber Ridge Trl.

Spruce Flats Branch

Buckhorn
Gap

Meigs Mtn. Trl.

considered commercially valuable in the early 20th century and were left to become the giants of the forest they are today. The final climb, at mile 3.3, signals your impending arrival at Buckhorn Gap, at mile 3.4. You'll intersect Meigs Mountain Trail, which goes to Elkmont, and Lumber Ridge Trail, which goes to Tremont.

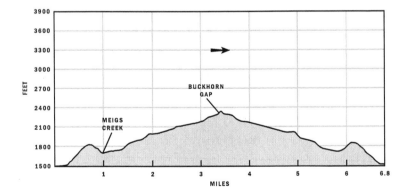

DIRECTIONS: From the Sugarlands Visitor Center, drive 12 miles east on Little River Road to The Sinks parking area, on your left. Meigs Creek Trail starts at the rear of the parking area.

GPS Trailhead Coordinates	05 BUCKHORN GAP VIA MEIGS CREEK
Latitude:	N35° 40' 9.9"
Longitude:	W83° 39' 43.1"
UTM Zone (WGS 84):	17S
Easting:	0259040
Northing:	3950360

SCENERY: ☆ ☆ ☆ ☆	DISTANCE: *8 miles round-trip*
DIFFICULTY: ☆ ☆ ☆	HIKING TIME: *4.5 hours round-trip*
TRAIL CONDITIONS: ☆ ☆ ☆	OUTSTANDING FEATURES: *Limited views*
SOLITUDE: ☆ ☆ ☆ ☆	*from Blanket Mountain, ideal picnic spot*
CHILDREN: ☆ ☆	

This hike starts along noisy Jakes Creek and ends atop Blanket Mountain, site of a former fire tower. Despite forest encroachment, a high open glade persists and makes an ideal spot for a high-country picnic, at 4,600 feet atop old Smoky. Follow a railroad grade for most of your journey through this watershed of bygone logging and human settlement.

🚶🚶 Not far from the trailhead lived the park's last permanent lifetime human resident, Lem Ownby. He passed away in 1980, at the age of 91. When the park was formed, many residents deeded over their lands and then were given lifetime leases to live out their days in the mountains they cherished as their own.

The Jakes Creek Trail leaves the end of Jakes Creek Road, winding upward to meet Cucumber Gap Trail at 0.3 miles. Continue on the jeep road and pass through the Meigs Mountain Trail junction at 0.4 miles. The trail begins rising a bit more steadily, crossing Waterdog Branch then Newt Prong at mile 1.5. The trail narrows as you leave reforested cropland, switchbacking to the left, then parallels high above Jakes Creek again.

After crossing a couple of side branches, come to Jakes Creek Backcountry Campsite 27, at mile 2.5. Continue working your way to the head of the watershed to arrive at Jakes Gap and a trail intersection, at mile 3.3. To your left, Miry Ridge travels 4.9 miles to the Appalachian Trail. Turn right and trace the now closed but still traveled Blanket Mountain Trail.

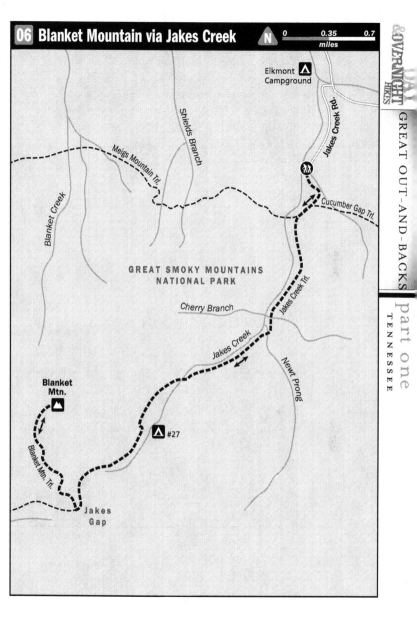

N

0   0.35   0.7
miles

Elkmont
Campground

Jakes Creek Rd.

Shields Branch

Meigs Mountain Trl.

Cucumber Gap Trl.

Blanket Creek

GREAT SMOKY MOUNTAINS
NATIONAL PARK

Jakes Creek Trl.

Cherry Branch

Jakes Creek

Newt Prong

Blanket
Mtn.

#27

Blanket Mtn. Trl.

Jakes
Gap

As you wind your way up to the summit of Blanket Mountain, where a surveyor once hung a blanket to delineate Indian lands, pass a rock outcrop on your left. Step atop the rocks and peer westward over nearby parkland. Just beyond the outcrop, at mile 4, you will come to the summit of Blanket Mountain. The remains of the fire tower and cabin make a good table and backrest for the weary and hungry hiker. Blanket Mountain is an idyllic place to laze away a summer's day while escaping the heat of the lowlands.

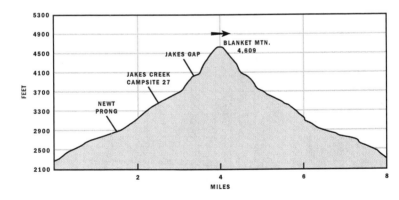

DIRECTIONS: Drive 4.9 miles on Little River Road from the Sugarlands Visitor Center to Elkmont. Turn left and follow the road 1.3 miles till you reach Elkmont Campground. Turn left at the sign for the Little River and Jakes Creek trailheads. Drive 0.5 miles, then follow the right fork 0.5 miles to its end at a parking area. Jakes Creek Trail starts at the left rear of the parking area.

GPS Trailhead Coordinates	06 BLANKET MOUNTAIN VIA JAKES CREEK
Latitude:	N35° 38' 45.1"
Longitude:	W83° 34' 58.4"
UTM Zone (WGS 84):	17S
Easting:	0266140
Northing:	3947530

07 Silers Bald

SCENERY: ✿ ✿ ✿ ✿ ✿	DISTANCE: *9.6 miles round-trip*
DIFFICULTY: ✿ ✿ ✿	HIKING TIME: *5 hours round-trip*
TRAIL CONDITIONS: ✿ ✿ ✿ ✿	OUTSTANDING FEATURES: *High country,*
SOLITUDE: ✿ ✿ ✿	*views all along hike, Silers Bald*
CHILDREN: ✿ ✿	

This hike fairly exudes the aura of the high country, as you traverse in and out of the spruce–fir forest that cloaks only the highest mantles of this land. Straddle the very spine of the state-line ridge, which offers windswept vistas into both Tennessee and North Carolina. Once you've reached the top of Silers Bald, you can look back and see where you started—Clingmans Dome parking area.

🚶 Start your hike on Forney Ridge Trail, leaving from the Clingmans Dome parking area. At mile 0.1 veer right on Clingmans Dome Bypass Trail. After a moderate climb to mile 0.6, you'll intersect the Appalachian Trail near Mount Buckley (elevation 6,500 feet). Continue west on the A.T., descending through an old burned-over section with views. Drop into a saddle then briefly ascend to a rock outcrop that makes a wonderful bench. Sit awhile and look far into North Carolina.

Enter the spruce–fir forest again, moving downward all the while. It is nearly always wet and cool here, pungent with the aroma of rich earth and growing and decaying vegetation. After a brief level section, come to the Goshen Prong Trail junction at mile 2.7. Continue your descent on the A.T. to arrive at the Double Springs Gap Trail shelter at mile 3.1. There's a small clearing in front of the shelter. As you arrive, there is a spring to your left, in North Carolina; this is the easiest place to obtain water.

Leave the shelter and climb Jenkins Knob, whose top is jumbled with beech trees. Beech leaves turn brown and often stay on the tree

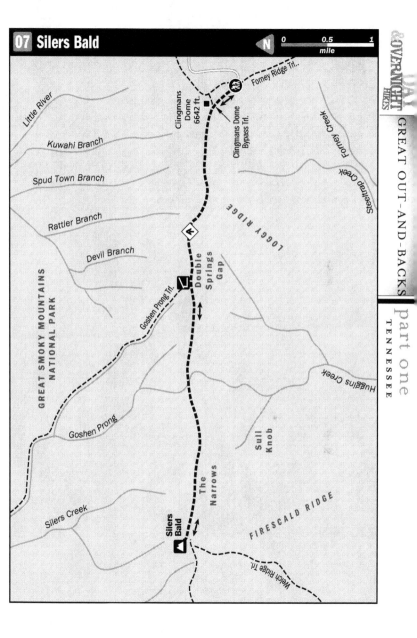

0   0.5   1
mile

N

Little River

Kuwahi Branch

Spud Town Branch

Rattler Branch

Devil Branch

GREAT SMOKY MOUNTAINS
NATIONAL PARK

Goshen Prong

Silers Creek

Goshen Prong Trl.

Double Springs Gap

The Narrows

Silers Bald

Clingmans Dome 6642 ft.

Clingmans Dome Bypass Trl.

Forney Ridge Trl.

Forney Creek

Steeltrap Creek

LOGGY RIDGE

Huggins Creek

Sull Knob

FIRESCALD RIDGE

Welch Ridge Trl.

throughout the winter, rattling in the wind. Below the knob you'll come to a field at mile 3.5. Welch Ridge lines the horizon to your right as you look into North Carolina. Pass through The Narrows, where the state-line ridge is barely wide enough for a footpath.

The Welch Ridge Trail junction intersects the A.T. at mile 4.4. Begin the final push to arrive atop Silers Bald (elevation 5,607 feet) at mile 4.8. Look back at the rugged crest of the Smokies. As you arrive at Silers Bald, a small side trail to your right allows long views into Tennessee. The A.T. continues down the shrinking bald to your left, which the park service is allowing to become reforested. Relax in what remains of the field and take it all in.

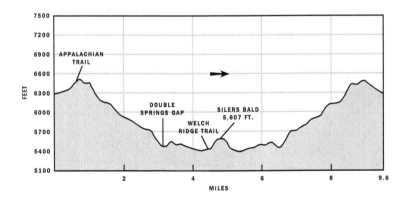

DIRECTIONS: From Newfound Gap, drive 7 miles to the end of Clingmans Dome Road. Forney Ridge Trail starts at the tip of the Clingmans Dome parking area.

GPS Trailhead Coordinates	07 SILERS BALD
Latitude:	N35° 33' 27.0"
Longitude:	W83° 29' 51.3"
UTM Zone (WGS 84):	17S
Easting:	0273640
Northing:	3937560

SCENERY: ✿ ✿ ✿ ✿
DIFFICULTY: ✿
TRAIL CONDITIONS: ✿ ✿ ✿ ✿ ✿
SOLITUDE: ✿ ✿ ✿ ✿ ✿
CHILDREN: ✿ ✿ ✿ ✿

DISTANCE: *6.4 miles round-trip*
HIKING TIME: *3.5 hours round-trip*
OUTSTANDING FEATURES: *Old homesites, small creeks, old steam engine*

Take a walk through time on this hike, which skirts the lower reaches of Mount LeConte, passing a collection of former farms and homesites that dot the Greenbrier area. The hike culminates at Injun Creek Backcountry Campsite, above which lies an old steam engine, a relic of the settler days in the Smokies. This isolated, historic walk is one of the most underrated and underused in the park.

Your hike starts on Grapeyard Ridge Trail, which follows a road once used by area settlers. You'll pass rock walls and more former roads that splinter off the trail. Ascend a small ridge and, at mile 0.6, you'll find an old homesite and the remains of a chimney. The trail follows a small brook leading to Rhododendron Creek. As you enter a former field, you will begin the first of several crossings of Rhododendron Creek and its tributaries, none of which are deep, though you may wet your boots a bit.

Wind up the creek valley, noting homesites on both sides of the trail. The 1931 topographic map of the Smokies shows 11 homesites in the Rhododendron Creek watershed. Rhododendron, the creek's namesake, constricts the path in areas near the creek, but the trail opens up away from water.

At mile 2.2, leave Rhododendron Creek and begin the ascent to James Gap. Another homesite sits in the saddle of James Gap at mile 2.8. Enter the Injun Creek watershed. As you descend, the inspiration for the name Injun Creek appears in a rivulet on your right. The body and wheels of a tractorlike steam engine

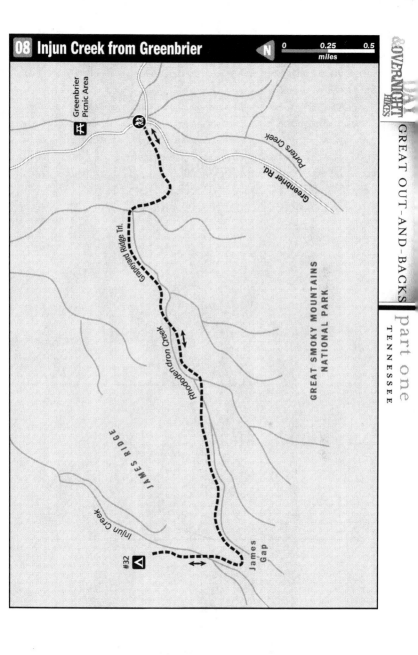

N

0   0.25   0.5
miles

Greenbrier Picnic Area

Greenbrier Rd.

Porters Creek

Grapeyard Ridge Trl.

Rhododendron Creek

GREAT SMOKY MOUNTAINS
NATIONAL PARK

JAMES RIDGE

Injun Creek

#32

James Gap

lie upturned, water running beneath the engine's rusted hulk.
A mapmaker mistakenly thought "Injun Creek" referred to Indians
rather than to this old steam engine that made its final turn in the
Smoky Mountains.

The road-turned-trail descends to reach the side trail to Injun
Creek Backcountry Campsite 32. Turn right on the side trail to the
camp at mile 3.2, where there is yet another homesite. Walk around
and look at the lasting changes the settlers made on the land, such as
creating level ground with rock-wall terraces. The campsite makes for
a good break spot. On your return journey, try to visualize how this
area will look once the forest reestablishes itself in this part of the
Smokies.

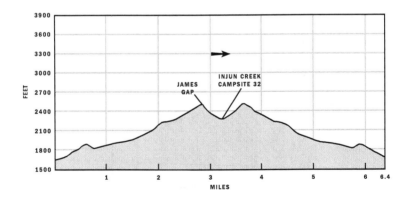

DIRECTIONS: From Gatlinburg, drive 6 miles east on US 321 to Greenbrier. Turn right at the Greenbrier sign and follow Greenbrier Road 3.1 miles to the intersection with Ramsey Prong Road, which crosses a bridge to your left. Park just before the intersection. Grapeyard Ridge Trail starts on the right side of Greenbrier Road.

GPS Trailhead Coordinates	08 INJUN CREEK FROM GREENBRIER
Latitude:	N35° 42' 25.8"
Longitude:	W83° 22' 57.2"
UTM Zone (WGS 84):	17S
Easting:	0284460
Northing:	3953830

09 Albright Grove

SCENERY: ✿ ✿ ✿ ✿	DISTANCE: 6.8 miles round-trip
DIFFICULTY: ✿ ✿	HIKING TIME: 3.25 hours round-trip
TRAIL CONDITIONS: ✿ ✿ ✿ ✿ ✿	OUTSTANDING FEATURES: Huge old-growth forest, pioneer cabin
SOLITUDE: ✿ ✿ ✿	
CHILDREN: ✿ ✿ ✿	

A hard-to-find trailhead keeps a lot of hikers off this trail. However, with good directions, it's a cinch. From the starting point, head up a wide bed on the Maddron Bald Trail, passing the Willis Baxter cabin, still intact after more than a century. Traverse a trail junction and start to climb a bit, then come to the side trail leading into Albright Grove. This nature trail loops through a giant forest of tulip trees, located between Dunn and Indian Camp creeks. The immensity of this woodland, named after the former National Park Service director Horace Albright, lures you to repeat the trek with friends in tow.

🥾 Pass around a pole gate and a trail sign. Head up an open trailbed beneath a second-growth deciduous forest that was once farmland. Remember the size of these trees, so you can compare them with their larger cousins up the path. The trail levels off and comes to the Willis Baxter cabin at 0.5 miles. This one-room cabin was built in 1889. Observe the notched logs at the corners of the cabin. Nearby you will find rock walls and a small, rocked-in spring. Developed springs are almost always found near old pioneer cabins and homesites because reliable water sources often lured homesteaders.

Continue up Maddron Bald Trail, coming to a trail junction at mile 1.2. Gabes Mountain Trail leaves left, and Old Settlers Trail departs right. History buffs can make a little side trip down Old Settlers Trail to see more homesites. Tree enthusiasts should continue on Maddron Bald Trail, which narrows and steepens a bit.

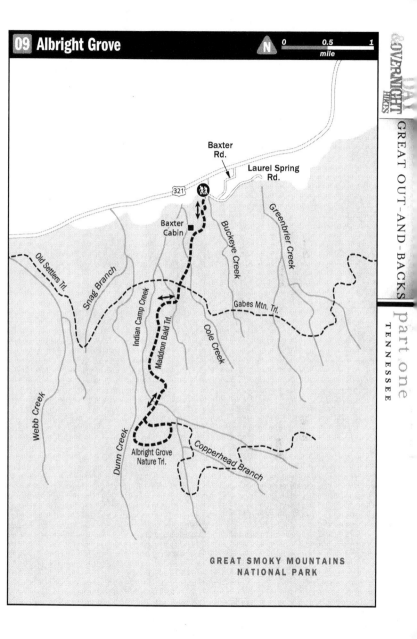

DAY
&OVERNIGHT
HIKES

GREAT OUT-AND-BACKS

part one

TENNESSEE

N

0   0.5   1
mile

Baxter
Rd.

Laurel Spring
Rd.

321

Baxter
Cabin

Buckeye Creek

Greenbrier Creek

Old Settlers Trl.

Snag Branch

Indian Camp Creek

Maddron Bald Trl.

Gabes Mtn. Trl.

Cole Creek

Webb Creek

Dunn Creek

Albright Grove
Nature Trl.

Copperhead Branch

GREAT SMOKY MOUNTAINS
NATIONAL PARK

Walk parallel to Indian Camp Creek and come to an old auto turnaround at mile 2.3. The path narrows yet again. Soon you will cross Indian Camp Creek and reach Albright Grove Nature Trail, at mile 2.9. Turn right here and revel in the land of the giants. Some of the grove's largest tulip trees have massive circumferences. There are other species here, such as Fraser magnolia, beech, and Carolina silverbell. Reach the end of the nature trail at mile 3.7. Turn back down Maddron Bald Trail. Your return trip will be 3.1 miles long.

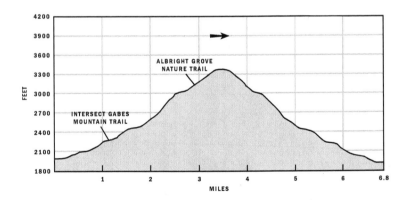

DIRECTIONS: Take US 321, East Parkway, north from Gatlinburg 15.6 miles to Baxter Road. (Baxter Road is just beyond Jellystone Park Campground and Smoky Mountain Creekside Rentals.) Turn right onto Baxter Road and follow it 0.3 miles to the gravel Laurel Springs Road. Veer sharply right onto Laurel Springs Road and follow it 100 yards to a pole gate and trail sign on the left. Maddron Bald Trail starts here.

GPS Trailhead Coordinates	09 ALBRIGHT GROVE
Latitude:	N35° 46' 9.9"
Longitude:	W83° 16' 1.2"
UTM Zone (WGS 84):	17S
Easting:	0295070
Northing:	3960510

10 Sutton Ridge Overlook

SCENERY: ✿ ✿ ✿ ✿

DIFFICULTY: ✿ ✿

TRAIL CONDITIONS: ✿ ✿ ✿ ✿ ✿

SOLITUDE: ✿ ✿ ✿ ✿

CHILDREN: ✿ ✿ ✿ ✿

DISTANCE: *3 miles round-trip*

HIKING TIME: *1.75 hours round-trip*

OUTSTANDING FEATURES: *Views, pioneer history*

This is a moderate hike to a great view. It's a wonder it's not hiked more. The walk starts near Cosby Campground and passes through pioneer lands that have long since been reforested. Cross a brook-trout stream while looking for signs of settlement, then climb a bit to Sutton Ridge. Take the side trail to a great view of the surrounding area. This hike is ideal for families that want to get off the beaten path, or for anyone who just wants a rewarding leg stretcher.

🚶🚶 Leave the Cosby hiker parking area and take Low Gap Trail. Cosby Creek lies to your left. Cruise through a forest of maple and buckeye. Pass the Cosby campground amphitheater and continue straight as Cosby Nature Trail forks left. Look for crumbled bits of pavement on this old road. Cross small streams on a series of footbridges. Cosby Nature Trail now comes in from the left. Low Gap Trail continues straight to a trail junction in a flat at 0.4 miles.

Turn left and follow Low Gap Trail just a few more steps to the beginning of Lower Mount Cammerer Trail. Continue straight on the latter as the Low Gap Trail forks right. Begin to look for evidence of settlers, such as rock walls and an old rocked-in spring. Tulip trees, which like to invade former fields, grow overhead. At mile 1.1, you'll come to Toms Creek. This stream is a brook-trout habitat. Brook trout are the only native Smokies trout and are normally relegated to higher-elevation streams because of past heavy stocking of rainbow and brown trout. But Toms Creek, at 2,500 feet, still sports brookies.

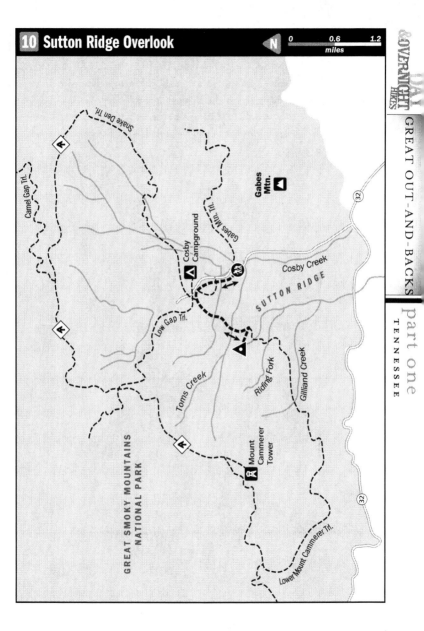

N

0   0.6   1.2
miles

Snake Den Trl.

Camel Gap Trl.

Gabes Mtn.

Gabes Mtn. Trl.

Cosby Campground

Cosby Creek

SUTTON RIDGE

Low Gap Trl.

Toms Creek

Riding Fork

Gilliand Creek

Mount Cammerer Tower

GREAT SMOKY MOUNTAINS NATIONAL PARK

Lower Mount Cammerer Trl.

32

32

After crossing Toms Creek on a footbridge, begin the short ascent to Sutton Ridge, reached at 1.4 miles. There is a horse hitch here. Turn right on the marked overlook trail and follow it 200 yards through woods of pine and oak to a clearing. Here, a splendid vista rewards hikers. To your left is the upper Cosby Valley. Gabes Mountain is the prominent mountain beyond Cosby Valley. Ahead is lower Cosby Valley, and to your right is Gililand Ridge on lower Mount Cammerer.

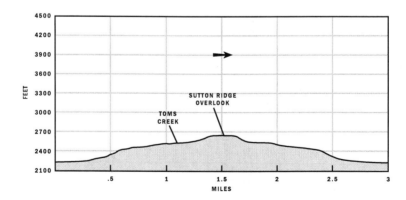

DIRECTIONS: From Gatlinburg, take US 321 north until it comes to a T-intersection with TN 32. Turn right on TN 32 and follow it a little more than a mile to the signed right turn into the Cosby section of the park. At 2.1 miles on Cosby Road, turn left into the hiker parking area. Low Gap Trail starts at the upper end of the parking area.

GPS Trailhead Coordinates	10 SUTTON RIDGE OVERLOOK
Latitude:	N35° 45' 28.0"
Longitude:	W83° 12' 31.0"
UTM Zone (WGS 84):	17S
Easting:	0300310
Northing:	3959130

II Brushy Mountain

SCENERY: ✿ ✿ ✿ ✿ ✿	DISTANCE: *11.4 miles round-trip*
DIFFICULTY: ✿ ✿ ✿	HIKING TIME: *5.5 hours round-trip*
TRAIL CONDITIONS: ✿ ✿ ✿ ✿	OUTSTANDING FEATURES: *Old homesites,*
SOLITUDE: ✿ ✿ ✿ ✿	*views from atop Brushy Mountain*
CHILDREN: ✿ ✿	

This hike traverses old farming areas and ascends through dry ridge country to arrive at Trillium Gap. A short climb leads you to the top of Brushy Mountain, where views await amid a heath-bald plant community. The more than 2,500-foot climb is steady, but the varied forest types and the view at the end are well worth the effort.

🚶🚶 Leave Greenbrier Road on Porters Creek Trail. The crashing Porters Creek will be your companion as you gently ascend, passing Ownby Cemetery about a half mile from the trailhead. The Brushy Mountain Trail junction is reached at mile I. Follow Brushy Mountain Trail as it leaves the junction at the far end of a loop and enters an old farm community in Porters Flat. Old rock walls, chimneys, and discarded metal items are all that remain of lives lived in the shadow of nearby Mount LeConte.

At mile 2.2, a small side trail leads down on your right to Fittified Spring, whose name is a first-rate example of mountain-folk vernacular (the spring has apparently steadied its flow since its naming). The trail passes near Long Branch but veers back south, leaving Porters Flat behind. The climb to Brushy Mountain remains steady as the trail enters pine-oak forest, prevalent on south-facing slopes.

At mile 3.1, a large boulder to your right offers a nice vista and rest spot. Continue climbing, and cross Trillium Branch twice. At mile 5.5, you'll reach grassy Trillium Gap. This is one of those

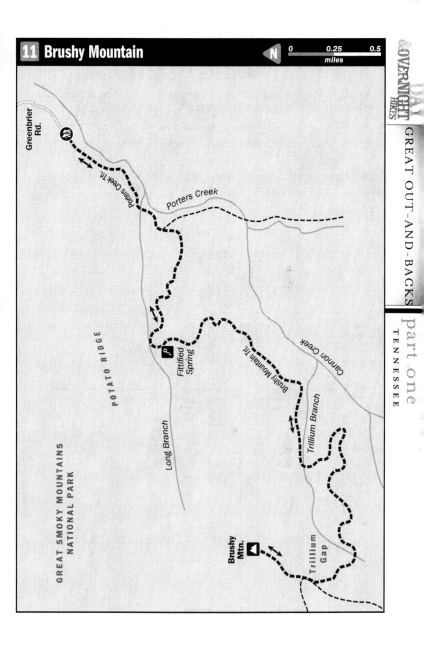

0   0.25   0.5
miles

Greenbrier Rd.

Porters Creek Trl

Porters Creek

POTATO RIDGE

Fittified Spring

Long Branch

Brushy Mountain Trl

Cannon Creek

Trillium Branch

GREAT SMOKY MOUNTAINS
NATIONAL PARK

Brushy Mtn.

Trillium Gap

mountain places with a perpetual cool breeze, demanding hikers stop to absorb the ambiance beneath the beech trees.

To reach the top of Brushy Mountain, veer right from the gap and follow the path beneath the tunnel of rhododendron and mountain laurel, which are the primary components of the heath–bald community. You'll come to an opening in the bald at mile 5.7. Brushy Mountain offers panoramas both above and below your 4,900-foot elevation. Above and to your south is the imposing bulk of Mount LeConte. To your east lies Porters Creek Valley, where you started. Below, to the north, are Gatlinburg and East Tennessee.

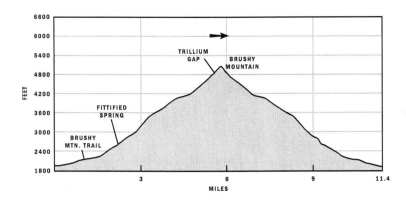

DIRECTIONS: From Gatlinburg, drive 6 miles on US 321. Turn right at the Greenbrier sign and drive 4 miles to the end of Greenbrier Road. Porters Creek Trail starts behind the parking area.

GPS Trailhead Coordinates	11 BRUSHY MOUNTAIN
Latitude:	N35° 41' 47.4"
Longitude:	W83° 23' 15.3"
UTM Zone (WGS 84):	17S
Easting:	0283960
Northing:	3952730

DAY &OVERNIGHT HIKES

GREAT OUT-AND-BACKS

part one

TENNESSEE

12 Mount Cammerer *via Low Gap*

SCENERY: ✿ ✿ ✿ ✿ ✿	DISTANCE: *10.8 miles round-trip*
DIFFICULTY: ✿ ✿ ✿	HIKING TIME: *5.25 hours round-trip*
TRAIL CONDITIONS: ✿ ✿ ✿	OUTSTANDING FEATURES: *Historic fire tower,*
SOLITUDE: ✿ ✿ ✿ ✿	*views from atop Mount Cammerer*
CHILDREN: ✿ ✿	

Formerly called White Rock by Tennesseans and Sharp Top by Carolinians, this mountaintop rock outcrop was renamed by the park service after Arno B. Cammerer, a former director of the National Park Service. No matter the name, this peak has incredible panoramas from its place on the Smokies crest. A historic wood-and-stone fire tower, long in disuse, has been repaired by the Friends of the Smokies. The restoration makes Mount Cammerer an even more desirable destination.

🥾 The trek to Cammerer starts in Cosby at the hiker parking area on Low Gap Trail. Follow the newer path, which skirts the campground 0.3 miles to the old Low Gap Trail, once maintained as a road to the fire tower. Enter farmland-turned-woodland to cross Cosby Creek on a footbridge at mile 0.9.

The trail begins a steady but not too steep climb toward the Smokies crest. The wide roadbed allows you to look around without having to watch your every step. At mile 1.3, the trail makes the first of several switchbacks amid a nearly virgin forest. Cross Cosby Creek (now tiny) again at mile 2.5, as the trail works its way toward Low Gap, where it meets the Appalachian Trail at mile 2.9.

At Low Gap, turn left on the A.T. and resume your ascent. This section of the A.T. is much less used than is the section near Newfound Gap. After a mile of steady climbing, the A.T. levels out near Sunup Knob, at mile 3.9. The trail is as level as trails come in the Smokies, rising slightly near the junction with Mount Cammerer Trail at mile 4.9.

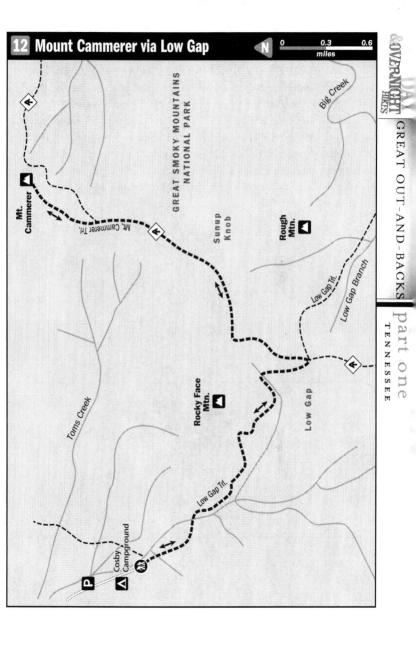

GREAT SMOKY MOUNTAINS
NATIONAL PARK

0   0.3   0.6
miles

N

Mt. Cammerer

Mt. Cammerer Trl.

Sunup Knob

Rough Mtn.

Low Gap Trl.

Low Gap Branch

Big Creek

Rocky Face Mtn.

Low Gap

Toms Creek

Low Gap Trl.

Cosby Campground

P

Turn left on Mount Cammerer Trail and follow the spur ridge out of the wooded junction into an area dominated by mountain laurel. After a slight dip, you'll reach the outcrop and tower at mile 5.4. Though it does enhance the setting, you don't need to climb the restored tower to enjoy the vistas from the jutting rocks, for you can see in every direction from the outcrop. The rock cut of Interstate 40 is visible to your east. Mount Sterling and its fire tower are to your south. In the foreground to the north is the appropriately named Stone Mountain and the hills of East Tennessee wave into the horizon. Maybe a place this spectacular does deserve three names.

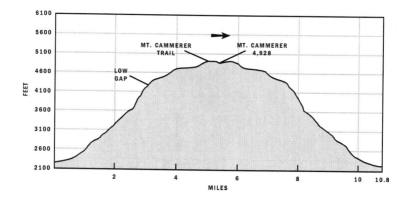

DIRECTIONS: From Gatlinburg, take US 321 east until it comes to a T-intersection with TN 32. Turn right on TN 32 and follow it a little more than a mile, turning right into the signed Cosby section of the park. At 2.1 miles, come to the hiker parking area to the left of the campground registration hut. Low Gap Trail starts in the upper corner of the parking area.

GPS Trailhead Coordinates	12 MOUNT CAMMERER VIA LOW GAP
Latitude:	N35° 45' 28.0"
Longitude:	W83° 12' 31.0"
UTM Zone (WGS 84):	17S
Easting:	0300310
Northing:	3959130

13 Mount Sterling *via Mount Sterling Gap*

SCENERY: ✿ ✿ ✿ ✿ ✿	DISTANCE: *5.6 miles round-trip*
DIFFICULTY: ✿ ✿	HIKING TIME: *2.75 hours round-trip*
TRAIL CONDITIONS: ✿ ✿ ✿ ✿ ✿	OUTSTANDING FEATURES: *Excellent views*
SOLITUDE: ✿ ✿ ✿ ✿	*from Mount Sterling tower*
CHILDREN: ✿ ✿ ✿	

At 5,842 feet, the top of Mount Sterling is adorned with one of only two original fire towers that hikers can climb to capture panoramas above the treetops. And the views from the spruce—fir high country of Sterling are limited only by the weather. The hike begins at Mount Sterling Gap and follows a short but sloping old jeep road to Mount Sterling Ridge and the high country. From the ridgetop, a short climb takes you to the tower.

🚶 Leave Mount Sterling Gap (elevation 3,890 feet) and begin climbing steeply up the wooded mountainside. The trail levels out a bit as it comes to an open area and Long Bunk Trail junction at mile 0.4. Resume climbing and make a sharp switchback to the right at mile 0.7.

The climb doesn't slacken much as it switchbacks farther up the mountain until it reaches the Mount Sterling Ridge Trail junction in a small grassy area at mile 2.3. The trail has now climbed 1,600 feet. Turn right at the junction, staying on the Mount Sterling Trail. Hike through forested and grassy areas, then pass a horse-hitch rack just before arriving at the top of Mount Sterling at mile 2.8. The mountaintop is also the location of Mount Sterling Backcountry Campsite 38.

The tower is at the crest of the mountain. Baxter Creek Trail, which comes from Big Creek Ranger Station, also ends at the tower. If you are thirsty, you'll find a spring on a side trail, a half mile down

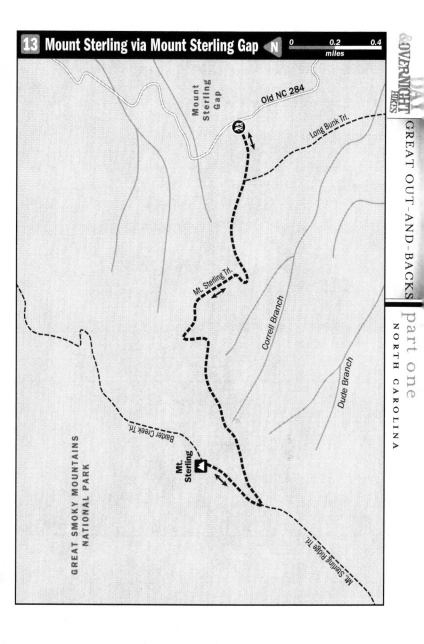

13 Mount Sterling via Mount Sterling Gap

N

0   0.2   0.4
miles

DAY &OVERNIGHT HIKES

GREAT OUT-AND-BACKS

part one

NORTH CAROLINA

Mount
Sterling
Gap

Old NC 284

Long Bunk Trl.

Mt. Sterling Trl.

Correll Branch

Dude Branch

Baxter Creek Trl.

Mt.
Sterling

GREAT SMOKY MOUNTAINS
NATIONAL PARK

Mt. Sterling Ridge Trl.

Baxter Creek Trail to your left (don't forget to treat the water). The park's eastern edge is the featured view from the tower. The main crest of the Smokies lies to the north. To the east, Interstate 40 cuts through the Pigeon River gorge. In the summer, the grassy area below the tower is an ideal lunch spot.

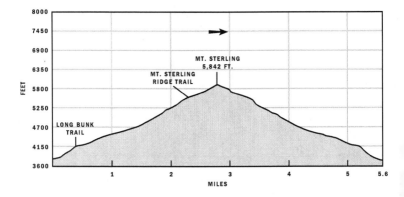

DIRECTIONS: From I-40, take exit 451, for Waterville. Cross the Pigeon River before turning left to follow it upstream. At an intersection 2.3 miles after crossing the Pigeon River, turn left on old NC 284 in Mount Sterling Village. Follow the dirt road 7 miles to Mount Sterling Gap. Mount Sterling Trail starts on your right at the gap.

GPS Trailhead Coordinates	13 MOUNT STERLING VIA MOUNT STERLING GAP
Latitude:	N35° 42' 0.7"
Longitude:	W83° 5' 52.0"
UTM Zone (WGS 84):	17S
Easting:	0310200
Northing:	3952510

14 Little Cataloochee Church

SCENERY: ✿ ✿ ✿ ✿
DIFFICULTY: ✿ ✿
TRAIL CONDITIONS: ✿ ✿ ✿ ✿
SOLITUDE: ✿ ✿ ✿ ✿ ✿
CHILDREN: ✿ ✿ ✿ ✿

DISTANCE: *7.6 miles round-trip*
HIKING TIME: *3.75 hours round-trip*
OUTSTANDING FEATURES: *Multiple historic homesites, Little Cataloochee Church*

The hike to Little Cataloochee Baptist Church traverses a historic mountain valley setting left over from the last century. Starting on Pretty Hollow Gap Trail, you'll hike past old fields and evidence of settlement before turning on Little Cataloochee Trail. Then you'll climb to Davidson Gap and into the Little Cataloochee Valley, with its many old homesites, to finally end up at the church, a fine structure built in 1890 and maintained to this day.

🚶 Leave Cataloochee Road and pass the Cataloochee horse camp at mile 0.2. Hike by some old fields, known locally as Indian Flats because Indians were there when the pioneers first arrived in this watershed. Come to the Little Cataloochee Trail junction at mile 0.7. Bear right on Little Cataloochee Trail, here an old roadbed, to head for Davidson Gap along Davidson Branch, which you'll cross several times.

Veer right up a tributary of Davidson Branch at mile 1.7. The trail steepens considerably, passing the remains of a settler's cabin on the left before reaching Davidson Gap at mile 2.3. Descend into the Little Cataloochee Valley, where more settlements were strung along Little Cataloochee Creek and its tributaries.

One tributary, Coggins Branch, will lead you into the valley. Of course, it has homesites of its own, marked by fence posts, rock walls, and old foundations, the most prominent of which is the Dan Cook place at mile 3. Built in 1856, the main house is deteriorating in the moist mountain climate, but the stone remnants of the barn are intact.

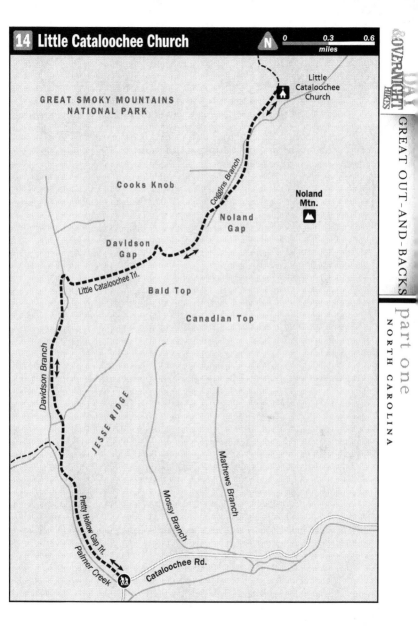

N

0   0.3   0.6
miles

GREAT SMOKY MOUNTAINS
NATIONAL PARK

Little
Cataloochee
Church

Cooks Knob

Coggins Branch

Noland
Mtn.

Noland
Gap

Davidson
Gap

Little Cataloochee Trl.

Bald Top

Canadian Top

Davidson Branch

JESSE RIDGE

Mossy Branch

Mathews Branch

Pretty Hollow Gap Trl.

Palmer Creek

Cataloochee Rd.

Pass more reminders of humanity's presence, coming to Little Cataloochee Church at mile 3.8. After you've passed so many dilapidated remains, the white church, well maintained by local families, looks even more impressive. There is a graveyard nearby.

The church makes a great base for further exploration of the entire valley and its historic settlements. Enjoy this hike into history in the Little Cataloochee Valley, but remember that the remnants are a living archaeological exhibit of life in the Smokies, and artifacts should be left where found.

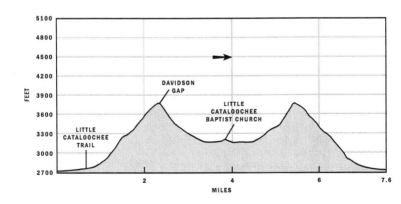

DIRECTIONS: Leave I-40 at exit 20 and get on NC 276. Drive
a short distance, then turn right on Cove Creek Road, following it
nearly 6 miles to enter the park. Two miles inside the park, turn
left onto Cataloochee Road. Follow it until it becomes gravel. Pretty
Hollow Gap Trail starts in a parking area on the right, just before
the gravel road crosses Palmer Creek.

GPS Trailhead Coordinates	14 LITTLE CATALOOCHEE CHURCH
Latitude:	N35° 37' 36.3"
Longitude:	W83° 6' 47.3"
UTM Zone (WGS 84):	17S
Easting:	0308660
Northing:	3944410

15 Hemphill Bald Hike

SCENERY: ✿ ✿ ✿ ✿ ✿	DISTANCE: 9.6 miles round-trip
DIFFICULTY: ✿ ✿ ✿	HIKING TIME: 5.5 hours round-trip
TRAIL CONDITIONS: ✿ ✿ ✿ ✿	OUTSTANDING FEATURES: Views from
SOLITUDE: ✿ ✿ ✿ ✿	Hemphill Bald, high-country hiking
CHILDREN: ✿ ✿	

This hike starts high and stays high most of the way as it skirts the park border on Cataloochee Divide. Its highest point, Hemphill Bald, offers great views. Most of the private-land side of the border remains open pasture, as much of the Smokies was a century ago, when Cataloochee Valley farmers would send their livestock to the hills to graze during the summer. The park service has let most of the Smokies balds reforest, and the contrast is striking, as you will find out along this hike.

🚶 Leave Polls Gap by hiking southeast on a singletrack path overlaying a wide railroad grade. Beech, birch, and cherry trees accompany the trail around Strawberry Knob. Reach the gap known as Sugartree Licks, then curve below Whim Knob. Look for misshapen old-growth yellow birch trees and large quartz boulders along the path. The trail reaches Garretts Gap and a fence line at 1.4 miles. This wooden split-rail fence delineates the park border for miles. Join Cataloochee Divide to ascend via several switchbacks, reaching Sheepback Knob at 3.1 miles.

The trail descends to an unnamed gap. A grassy road ends at the gap on the private-land side of the fence. The trail angles up the north side of no-longer-bald Little Bald Knob to regain the crest of Cataloochee Divide past the knob. A prolonged moderate downgrade in a young forest leads to Pine Tree Gap. The private side of the ridge, just across the fence from you, becomes open and grassy. The pastureland affords views of Hemphill Bald ahead, which is perfectly divided by the park border. You will reach Pine Tree Gap

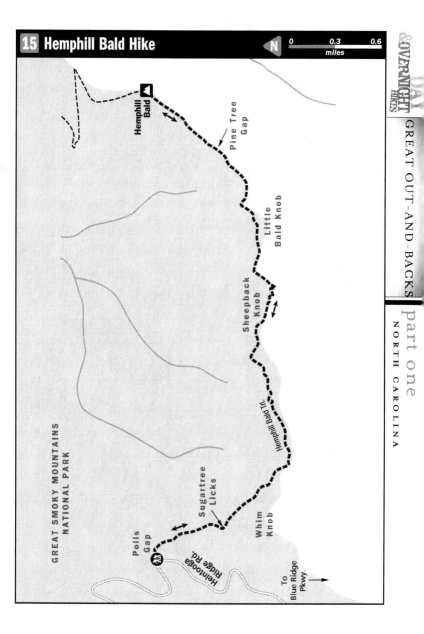

15 Hemphill Bald Hike

N

0   0.3   0.6
miles

GREAT OUT-AND-BACKS

part one
NORTH CAROLINA

Hemphill Bald

Pine Tree Gap

Little Bald Knob

Sheepback Knob

Hemphill Bald Trl.

Sugartree Licks

Whim Knob

Polls Gap

Heintooga Ridge Rd.

GREAT SMOKY MOUNTAINS NATIONAL PARK

To Blue Ridge Pkwy.

at 4.1 miles, where there are no pine trees. Begin the 300-foot climb to the top of Hemphill Bald. Views open to the southeast. The area is a study in reforestation and land management—where there is no grazing or mowing, the mountain has grown up with trees, despite the short growing season at this altitude. And with grazing and mowing, the bald of Hemphill Bald stays open and offers wonderful vistas.

You'll reach the top of the bald at 4.8 miles, where you'll find a stone table, hitching rack, and benches on the ranch just across the park border. A kiosk detailing all the mountains and towns to the east of Hemphill Bald is embedded in the table and provides insight into exactly what you are looking at. And it is a lot.

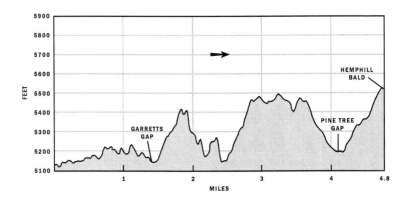

DIRECTIONS: From the Oconaluftee Visitor Center near Cherokee, take Newfound Gap Road 0.5 miles south to the Blue Ridge Parkway. Turn left onto the Blue Ridge Parkway and follow it 10.8 miles to Heintooga Ridge Road. Turn left on Heintooga Ridge Road and drive 6 miles to Polls Gap, on your right. Hemphill Bald Trail leaves right.

GPS Trailhead Coordinates	15 HEMPHILL BALD HIKE
Latitude:	N35° 33' 47.7"
Longitude:	W83° 9' 42.2"
UTM Zone (WGS 84):	17S
Easting:	0304080
Northing:	3937420

16 Flat Creek Falls

SCENERY: ☆ ☆ ☆ ☆ ☆	DISTANCE: 3.2 miles round-trip
DIFFICULTY: ☆ ☆	HIKING TIME: 2 hours round-trip
TRAIL CONDITIONS: ☆ ☆ ☆ ☆	OUTSTANDING FEATURES: View, waterfall,
SOLITUDE: ☆ ☆ ☆ ☆	attractive high-country woodland
CHILDREN: ☆ ☆ ☆ ☆	

This is the sort of route that makes hikers wonder, "Why aren't more people hiking this trail?" Maybe because Flat Creek Trail begins on a lesser-traveled road, or maybe because it has no other trail connections. For Smoky Mountain enthusiasts, there should be no maybes about hiking this path. It starts at more than 5,300 feet and passes a wonderful view of the Smokies' crest before entering a high-country forest of spruce and yellow birch. The path then descends along Flat Creek and makes its way to the highest elevation falls accessible by trail in the park. It is a fine family hike if you are careful to keep children under control around this steep and narrow cascade.

🥾🥾 Start the walk on Flat Creek Trail, swinging around Heintooga Picnic Area on the left. At 0.1 mile, near a water fountain, come to a cleared overlook. To the north is the crest of the Smokies. With binoculars you can see the Clingmans Dome tower. Continue straight and you'll soon come to a trail junction. Take the narrow path dropping down to the right. Overhead there are tall spruces and yellow birches. You'll soon work your way around the knob that once held Flat Creek Bald. It is forested now, though the understory remains grassy. Flat Creek is at 0.7 miles. You can easily cross the small stream on a footbridge.

Keep a fairly level course through a pleasant woodland, crossing Flat Creek twice more on footlogs, just beyond mile 1. Wet-weather drainages bisect the trailbed from the left as the trail moves away from the creek. You'll reach the side trail for Flat Creek Falls at mile 1.5. Turn right here and descend; the sound of rushing water

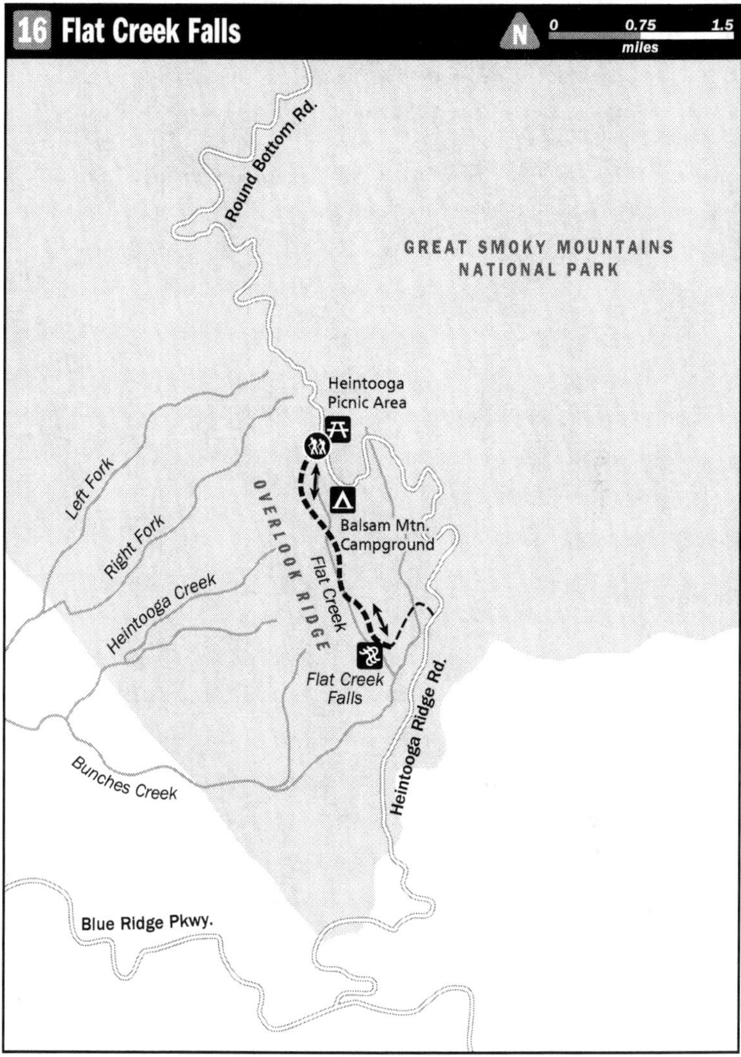
16 Flat Creek Falls
N
0
0.75
1.5
miles
Round Bottom Rd.
GREAT SMOKY MOUNTAINS
NATIONAL PARK
Heintooga
Picnic Area
Left Fork
Right Fork
OVERLOOK RIDGE
Balsam Mtn.
Campground
Flat Creek
Heintooga Creek
Flat Creek
Falls
Heintooga Ridge Rd.
Bunches Creek
Blue Ridge Pkwy.

becomes audible as you near the creek at mile 1.6. Closely supervise the kids in this area: Flat Creek puts gravity to use on its way to meet Bunches Creek in the valley below. There are views of the Bunches Creek watershed near Flat Creek. Side trails spur down toward the steep, narrow falls. It is challenging to get a complete view of the entire cascade because the fall is narrow and drops down a heavily vegetated rock chute. Nevertheless, stunning views abound, rewarding hikers for their trek.

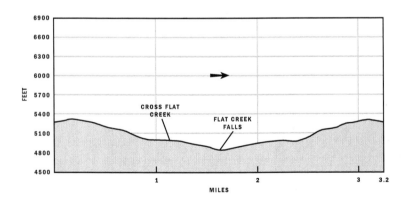

DIRECTIONS: From the Oconaluftee Visitor Center near
Cherokee, take Newfound Gap Road 0.5 miles south to the Blue
Ridge Parkway, where you'll turn left to follow the parkway
10.8 miles to Heintooga Ridge Road. Turn left on Heintooga Ridge
Road and go 8.7 miles to Heintooga Picnic Area. Flat Creek Falls
Trail starts at the end of the nearby auto turnaround.

GPS Trailhead Coordinates	16 FLAT CREEK FALLS
Latitude:	N35° 34' 24.1"
Longitude:	W83° 10' 49.4"
UTM Zone (WGS 84):	17S
Easting:	0302420
Northing:	3938590

17 Andrews Bald

SCENERY: ✿ ✿ ✿ ✿ ✿
DIFFICULTY: ✿
TRAIL CONDITIONS: ✿ ✿ ✿ ✿
SOLITUDE: ✿ ✿
CHILDREN: ✿ ✿ ✿ ✿ ✿

DISTANCE: *3.6 miles round-trip*
HIKING TIME: *1.75 hours round-trip*
OUTSTANDING FEATURES: *Spruce–fir forest, Andrews Bald*

This is one of the Smokies' finest hikes. The trip passes through an extraordinary spruce–fir forest to the grassy field of Andrews Bald. Resplendent with stunning views, this is an ideal backdrop for a picnic in the sky. Andrews Bald is one of only two grassy fields in the Smokies that the park service maintains in their "original" state. The origin of these fields is not clear, although natural fires, clearing by Indians, and grazing cattle possibly kept the fields clear.

🚶🚶 After leaving the Clingmans Dome parking area on Forney Ridge Trail, you zigzag through an evergreen forest reminiscent of Maine or Canada. At 0.1 mile into the hike, make sure you veer left, away from Clingmans Dome Bypass Trail. Forney Ridge Trail descends along a rocky section that allows views to the south and, at mile 1, intersects Forney Creek Trail.

Continue along the undulating and rocky ridge to arrive at the southern end of Andrews Bald at mile 1.8. The lush grassy field (elevation 5,800 feet) beckons you to lie down, but that would deny you the expansive views of the southern range of the Smokies and beyond, as far south as the clarity of the sky allows. This bald, the Smokies' highest, also offers marvelous flower displays in June and blueberries and blackberries in late summer.

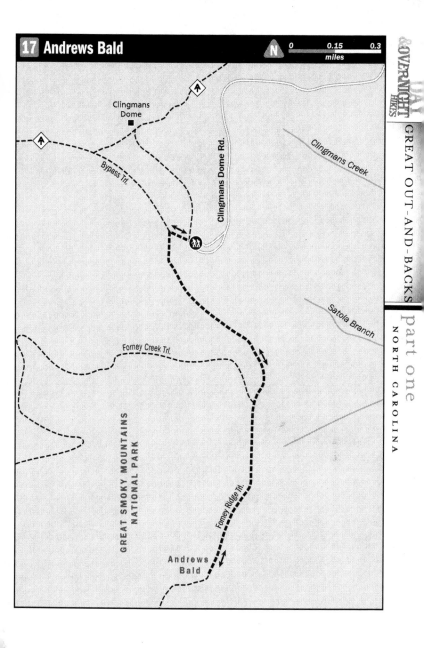

N

0   0.15   0.3
miles

Clingmans Dome

Clingmans Creek

Bypass Trl.

Clingmans Dome Rd.

Satola Branch

Forney Creek Trl.

GREAT SMOKY MOUNTAINS NATIONAL PARK

Forney Ridge Trl.

Andrews Bald

DIRECTIONS: From Newfound Gap, drive 7 miles to the end of
Clingmans Dome Road. Forney Ridge Trail starts at the tip of the
Clingmans Dome parking area.

GPS Trailhead Coordinates   17 ANDREWS BALD
Latitude: N35° 33' 27.0"
Longitude: W83° 29' 51.3"
UTM Zone (WGS 84):   17S
Easting: 0273640
Northing: 3937560

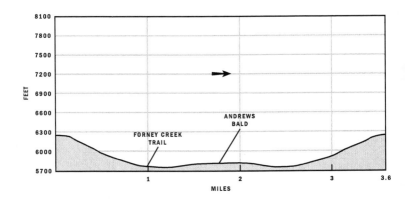

18 Shuckstack *from Twentymile Ranger Station*

SCENERY: ✿ ✿ ✿ ✿ ✿	DISTANCE: *10.2 miles round-trip*
DIFFICULTY: ✿ ✿ ✿	HIKING TIME: *5.25 hours round-trip*
TRAIL CONDITIONS: ✿ ✿ ✿ ✿ ✿	OUTSTANDING FEATURES: *Waterfall, views*
SOLITUDE: ✿ ✿ ✿ ✿	*from Shuckstack Mountain*
CHILDREN: ✿ ✿	

Twentymile is one of the Smokies' most remote areas. You'll travel along Twentymile Creek on an old railroad grade, past Twentymile Cascades, up to the Appalachian Trail and Shuckstack Mountain, and finally to a fire tower that offers one of those worth-the-effort, above-the-treetops, 360-degree panoramas.

🏃🏃 Begin your hike at the gated road on the Twentymile Trail. Pass a park service barn in a clearing on your right. Cross Moore Spring Branch on a wide bridge at mile 0.6. On the far side of the bridge is the Wolf Ridge Trail junction. Bear right, staying on Twentymile Trail. At mile 0.7, a sign marks the side trail to the bottom of Twentymile Cascades. Take the side trail for a view of the creek dropping over a series of wide stone slabs.

Return to the main trail, ascending gradually. Cross Twentymile Creek on wide bridges at miles 1.4 and 1.6. Come to Twentymile Creek Backcountry Campsite 93, at mile 1.7. Immediately cross another bridge beyond the campsite. The trail now runs farther above the creek, passing over tributary streams, only to cross Twentymile Creek twice more on bridges before arriving at Proctor Gap and a trail junction at mile 3.

Bear right at the trail junction, staying on Twentymile Trail and enjoying its steady grade. The trail now parallels Proctor Branch. At mile 3.5, the trail steepens, leaving Proctor Branch behind. The final ascent to the A.T. is completed in a series of switchbacks to arrive at Sassafras Gap at mile 4.7.

N 0   0.4   0.8
feet

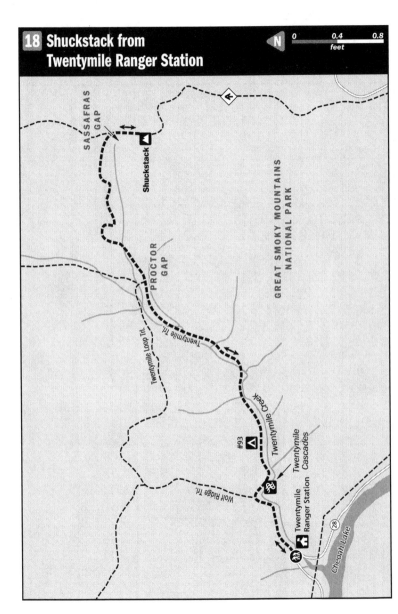

SASSAFRAS GAP

Shuckstack

PROCTOR GAP

GREAT SMOKY MOUNTAINS NATIONAL PARK

Twentymile Loop Trl.

Twentymile Trl.

Twentymile Creek

Wolf Ridge Trl.

#93

Twentymile Cascades

Twentymile Ranger Station

28

Cheoah Lake

Turn right on the A.T., climbing out of Sassafras Gap, and come to a side trail on top of Shuckstack at mile 5. Turn left and climb a steep grade 0.1 mile to the top of Shuckstack and a fire tower (elevation 4,020 feet). Atop the tower, views abound. The main crest of the Smokies is northward. Fontana Lake covers the flooded valley of the Little Tennessee River to the southeast. From this vantage point, the surrounding Southern Appalachian sea of mountains looks especially rugged.

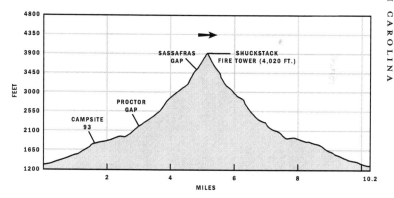

DIRECTIONS: From Townsend, Tennessee, take US 321 north to
Foothills Parkway. Follow Foothills Parkway west to US 129. Follow
US 129 south into North Carolina. Turn left on NC 28. Follow
NC 28, driving 2.6 miles to Twentymile Ranger Station, on your
left. Park beyond the ranger station and walk up to the gated road
to begin your hike on Twentymile Trail. From the courthouse in
Bryson City, North Carolina, take US 19 south 5.4 miles to NC 28.
Drive 30 miles down NC 28 to reach Twentymile Ranger Station,
which will be on your right.

GPS Trailhead Coordinates	18 SHUCKSTACK FROM TWENTYMILE RANGER STATION
Latitude:	N35° 28' 9.9"
Longitude:	W83° 52' 18.8"
UTM Zone (WGS 84):	17S
Easting:	0239350
Northing:	3928700

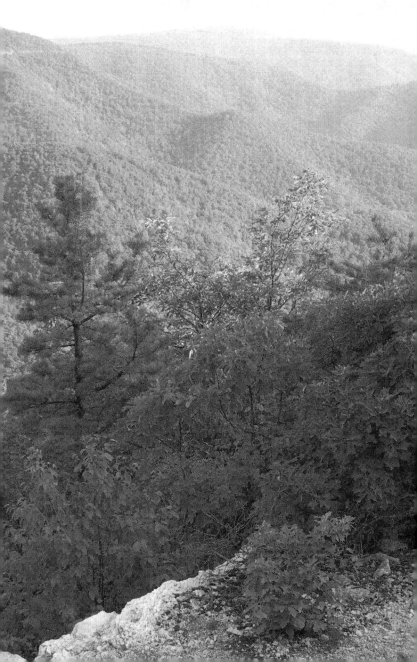

part two
GREAT DAY LOOPS

2

The return
trip to the
AT will
get you
huffing and
puffing,
which
thinking of
all the
people that
skipped
this
second view
as
evidenced
by the
much less
used trail
tread.

19 Pine Mountain Loop

SCENERY: ✿ ✿ ✿ ✿	DISTANCE: *7.9 miles*
DIFFICULTY: ✿ ✿ ✿	HIKING TIME: *4 hours*
TRAIL CONDITIONS: ✿ ✿ ✿ ✿	OUTSTANDING FEATURES: *Pine-oak forest,*
SOLITUDE: ✿ ✿ ✿ ✿	*Abrams Creek*
CHILDREN: ✿ ✿ ✿	

The two Abrams Creek ford crossings account for this hike's difficulty rating. The first ford might be avoided, especially during the summer months when the footlog is restored after winter rains. The second ford is the toughest in the park. But don't let the fords discourage you from taking this scenic loop hike. It is a good opportunity to explore the pine- and oak-forested western end of the park in a less-peopled setting. Leave Abrams Creek Ranger Station to cross Abrams Creek for the first time. Then wind up Pine Mountain on a jeep road, descending into Scott Gap. Next, work your way down a south slope to cross the creek again. Follow Abrams Creek on the narrow, twisting Little Bottoms Trail to return to the ranger station via Cooper Road.

🥾 Start your hike by walking from the parking area back toward Abrams Creek Ranger Station. Rabbit Creek Trail starts at the upper end of the horse pasture. Follow Rabbit Creek Trail to the first crossing of Abrams Creek at 0.1 mile. Look downstream for the footlog. If it's not there, you'll have to ford the creek. After crossing Abrams Creek, immediately enter an old homesite, with reforesting fields and an old chimney. Start climbing Pine Mountain, switching back at the point of a ridge. Top out on Pine Mountain at mile 2, then descend to Scott Gap and a trail junction at mile 2.5.

Scott Gap campsite 16 and a spring are down the trail to your right. Turn left at the gap on Hannah Mountain Trail, which follows south slopes on its descent to Abrams Creek, with many laurel bushes and several pine trees along the route. The second Abrams Creek crossing is at mile 4.3. This is a ford for sure. Use trekking

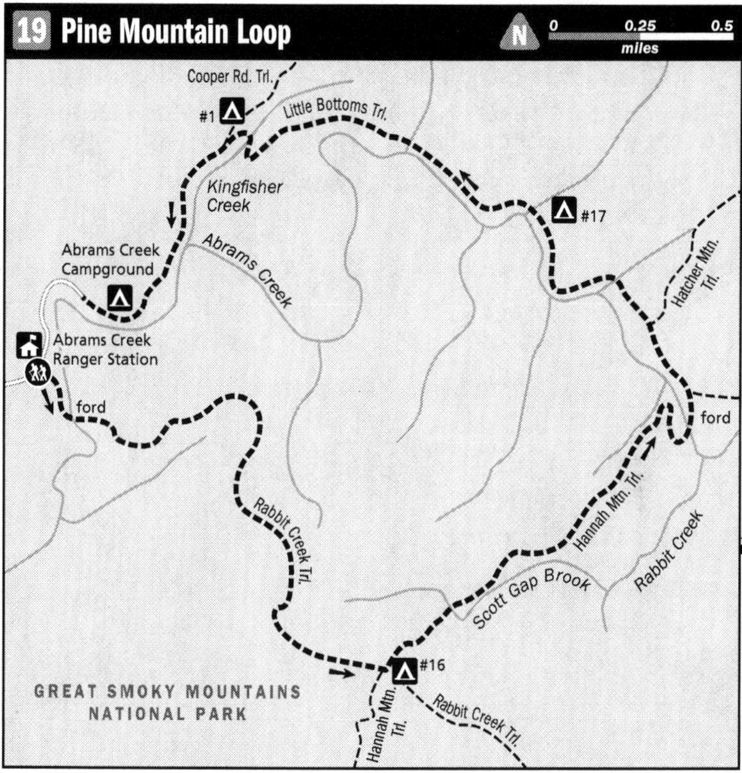
19 Pine Mountain Loop
N
0
0.25
0.5
miles
Cooper Rd. Trl.
#1
Little Bottoms Trl.
Kingfisher Creek
Abrams Creek Campground
Abrams Creek
#17
Hatcher Mtn. Trl.
Abrams Creek Ranger Station
ford
ford
Hannah Mtn. Trl.
Rabbit Creek Trl.
Rabbit Creek
Scott Gap Brook
#16
GREAT SMOKY MOUNTAINS NATIONAL PARK
Hannah Mtn. Trl.
Rabbit Creek Trl.

poles or find a stout branch for balance and face upstream as you ford.

Once across, you'll come to Hatcher Mountain Trail junction. Turn left on Hatcher Mountain Trail and climb a short distance to another trail junction at mile 4.5. Turn left again and follow Little Bottoms Trail, which winds far above the Abrams Creek gorge only to drop down to creek level at Little Bottoms Backcountry

Campsite 17, at mile 5.3.

The trail snakes along the creek then leaves the gorge to top a side ridge at mile 6.5. Wind along a pair of switchbacks, and you'll be down at Kingfisher Creek and the Cooper Road Trail junction at mile 6.8. Turn left on Cooper Road Trail to arrive at the Abrams Creek campground at mile 7.9. The parking area is 0.5 miles farther down Abrams Creek Road.

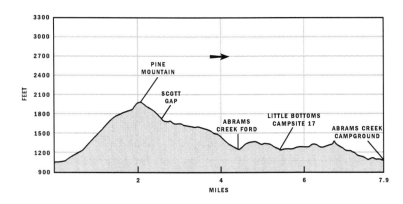

DIRECTIONS: From Townsend, Tennessee, drive west on US 321 and turn left onto Foothills Parkway. Follow Foothills Parkway west to US 129, and turn left onto US 129 at Chilhowee Lake. Head south 0.5 miles to Happy Valley Road. Turn left on Happy Valley Road, following it 6 miles to Abrams Creek Road. Turn right on Abrams Creek Road and drive I mile to the campground, passing the ranger station. Cooper Road Trail starts behind the campground. Park your car in the designated area near the ranger station.

GPS Trailhead Coordinates	19 PINE MOUNTAIN LOOP
Latitude:	N35° 36' 35.4"
Longitude:	W83° 56' 8.6"
UTM Zone (WGS 84):	17S
Easting:	0234072
Northing:	3944436

20 Rich Mountain Loop

SCENERY: ✿ ✿ ✿ ✿	DISTANCE: *8.5 miles*
DIFFICULTY: ✿ ✿	HIKING TIME: *4.25 hours*
TRAIL CONDITIONS: ✿ ✿ ✿ ✿ ✿	OUTSTANDING FEATURES: *Old cabin,*
SOLITUDE: ✿ ✿ ✿	*view of Cades Cove and mountains beyond*
CHILDREN: ✿ ✿ ✿	

This is a pleasant day hike that shows Cades Cove from a unique perspective, with a stop by the historic John Oliver cabin thrown in for good measure. Initially you'll stay in the basin of the cove then climb up Rich Mountain to an inspiring overlook. After you top out on Rich Mountain, with good but interspersed views, you'll circle back down on Crooked Arm Ridge Trail, completing the loop.

🏃 Start your hike on Rich Mountain Loop Trail, rock-hopping over Crooked Arm Branch, then come to a trail junction at mile 0.5. This is the return point of your loop. Veer left on Rich Mountain Loop Trail. Cross Harrison Branch as you continue northwestward. At mile 1.2, the John Oliver cabin, built in 1820, will be on your left. Oliver was an early settler of the cove and helped populate it with his many offspring.

The climb begins in earnest when you turn up Martha's Branch and begin switchbacking up Rich Mountain, along Cave Ridge. Your first notable view of the cove opens up on your left at mile 3, just as you come to the 3,000-foot level. The Indian Grave Gap Trail junction is at mile 3.4 and offers another cove view.

Turn right and begin a moderate climb on Indian Grave Gap Trail, reaching Rich Mountain Trail junction at mile 4.2. Push on up Indian Grave Gap Trail near the top of Rich Mountain, where a fire tower once stood near the spur trail to your left. The forest cover limits the views now, but the clearing makes an ideal picnic spot.

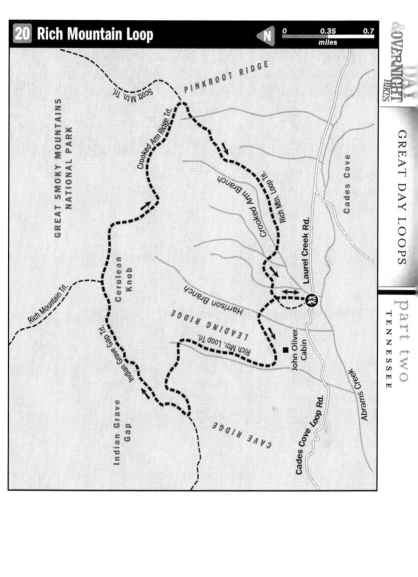

N

0   0.35   0.7
miles

PINKROOT RIDGE

Scott Mtn. Trl.

Crooked Arm Ridge Trl.

GREAT SMOKY MOUNTAINS
NATIONAL PARK

Cades Cove

Crooked Arm Branch

Rich Mtn. Loop

Laurel Creek Rd.

Rich Mountain Trl.

Cerulean Knob

Harrison Branch

LEADING RIDGE

Rich Mtn. Loop Trl.

John Oliver
Cabin

Indian Grave Gap Trl.

Indian Grave Gap

CAVE RIDGE

Cades Cove Loop Rd.

Abrams Creek

Start descending Rich Mountain. At mile 5.9, near a clearing for a power line, is the junction with Crooked Arm Ridge Trail. As you begin the trail, keep your eyes raised to enjoy the vista from an overlook. Switchback down toward Cades Cove, crossing Crooked Arm Branch near the base of the mountain.

Complete the loop at mile 8, where the trail intersects Rich Mountain Loop Trail. Follow it 0.5 miles back down to the loop road and to the cove you just viewed from above.

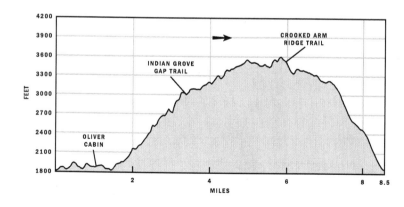

DIRECTIONS: From the Townsend "Wye," turn right onto Laurel Creek Road, and follow it 7.4 miles to the beginning of Cades Cove Loop Road. Park at the beginning of the loop and walk a short way down the loop road to Rich Mountain Loop Trail, which is on your right.

GPS Trailhead Coordinates	20 RICH MOUNTAIN LOOP
Latitude:	N35° 36' 25.6"
Longitude:	W83° 47' 13.6"
UTM Zone (WGS 84):	17S
Easting:	0247500
Northing:	3943710

21 Finley Cane Loop

SCENERY: ✿ ✿ ✿ ✿	DISTANCE: *8.9 miles*
DIFFICULTY: ✿ ✿	HIKING TIME: *4.25 hours*
TRAIL CONDITIONS: ✿ ✿ ✿ ✿	OUTSTANDING FEATURES: *Old homesites,*
SOLITUDE: ✿ ✿ ✿ ✿	*mountainsides, small creeks*
CHILDREN: ✿ ✿ ✿ ✿	

Although you must cross a road during this excursion, the trails on this hike are lightly used, offering a pleasantly undulating loop with very little climbing, considering the mountainous setting. First, you will walk among old homesites, the trail gently winding along the slope of Turkeypen Ridge. Then you'll follow an old road to the historic Bote Mountain Trail. Finally, Bote Mountain Trail will lead you to Finley Cane Trail along the northern base of Bote Mountain to complete your loop.

🏃 Start your hike along Turkeypen Ridge Trail, descending from Big Spring Cove to Crib Gap Trail junction at mile 0.2. Continue on Turkeypen Ridge Trail through an old homesite with relics scattered amid sparse woods. Leave Big Spring Cove to work your way up to a nearly level ridge extending from a flank of Scott Mountain. Follow the trail as it drops slightly to cross the most notable creek on the path, Pinkroot Branch, at mile 1.3.

Wind your way along Turkeypen Ridge and notice the differing forest types, determined by the amount of sun exposure. South-facing slopes include various species of pine and mountain laurel, whereas shaded ravines support rhododendron. The trail takes a northeastward course, sloping to reach Schoolhouse Gap Trail at mile 3.4.

Turn right on Schoolhouse Gap Trail as it parallels Spence Branch to Laurel Creek Road at mile 4.5. Turn left on the road, go 50 yards, and cross over to Bote Mountain Trail. Return to the

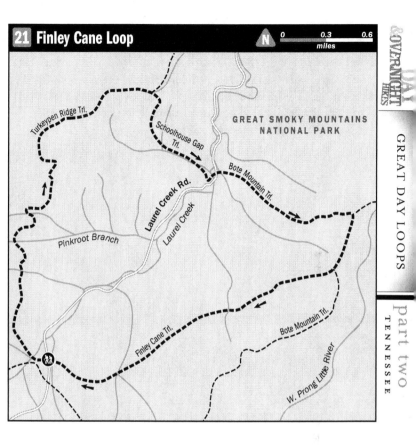

21 Finley Cane Loop

N   0   0.3   0.6
              miles

DAY & OVERNIGHT HIKES

GREAT DAY LOOPS

part two
TENNESSEE

GREAT SMOKY MOUNTAINS
NATIONAL PARK

Turkeypen Ridge Trl.

Schoolhouse Gap Trl.

Bote Mountain Trl.

Laurel Creek Rd.

Laurel Creek

Pinkroot Branch

Finley Cane Trl.

Bote Mountain Trl.

W. Prong Little River

woods up this former road. Like the Schoolhouse Gap road-turned-trail, this trail was once part of a plan to connect Maryville, Tennessee, to the Hazel Creek area.

Stay on Bote Mountain Trail as you pass West Prong Trail at mile 5.7. At mile 6.3, turn right for the final leg of your loop, Finley Cane Trail. The woodlands here feature tulip trees, sugar maples, and beeches. Pass Finley Cane's only patch of cane. Crossing many small rills running perpendicular to the trail, you'll hike in and out of watery hollows to a trail junction at mile 8.3. To the right, a horse trail passes under Laurel Creek Road to connect with Turkeypen Ridge Trail. Continue ahead on Finley Cane Trail to complete your loop to Laurel Creek Road and the Big Spring Cove parking area at mile 8.9.

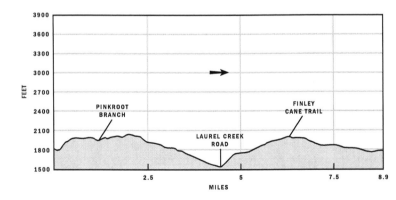

DIRECTIONS: From Townsend, Tennessee, drive east, turning left at the Townsend "Wye" onto Laurel Creek Road. Head 5.6 miles toward Cades Cove. Turkeypen Ridge Trail is on your right at the small Big Spring Cove parking area that extends along both sides of the road.

GPS Trailhead Coordinates	21 FINLEY CANE LOOP
Latitude:	N35° 37' 40.3"
Longitude:	W83° 43' 32.4"
UTM Zone (WGS 84):	17S
Easting:	0253110
Northing:	3945920

22 Spence Field–Russell Field Loop

SCENERY: ✿ ✿ ✿ ✿ ✿
DIFFICULTY: ✿ ✿ ✿
TRAIL CONDITIONS: ✿ ✿ ✿ ✿
SOLITUDE: ✿ ✿
CHILDREN: ✿ ✿

DISTANCE: *13 miles*
HIKING TIME: *6.75 hours*
OUTSTANDING FEATURES: *Views from Spence Field, Little Bald*

This strenuous all-day hike amply rewards those who want to see the Smokies from bottom to top. Starting in Cades Cove, climb along a deeply forested crashing mountain stream to ultimately intersect the main crest of the Smokies and the famed Appalachian Trail. Once on the A.T., you'll find outstanding views lie before you at Spence Field and Little Bald. Return to Cades Cove via Russell Field Trail with its section of old-growth trees.

🏃 Follow Anthony Creek Trail beyond the horse camp, bypassing Crib Gap Trail at 0.5 miles. Continue, making the first of four crossings of Anthony Creek and its tributaries. The bigger crossings offer footbridges for ease of travel. Just beyond the fourth creek crossing, you'll reach a trail junction at mile 1.3. This is where you'll return upon completing your loop. Trace Anthony Creek Trail, saving Russell Field Trail for the return journey. Continue climbing, passing Anthony Creek Backcountry Campsite 9, on your right at 2.7 miles. Shortly beyond the campsite, leave Anthony Creek and ascend to the intersection with Bote Mountain Trail at 3.3 miles. Turn right up Bote Mountain Trail along an old jeep road and continue to a turnaround at mile 4. The trail narrows and becomes a deeply rutted rocky path, ascending steadily through rhododendron to arrive at the lower reaches of Spence Field and the Appalachian Trail at 5.6 miles.

Take time to explore the former pasture that is growing over but still offers grand views of Fontana Lake in North Carolina and Cades

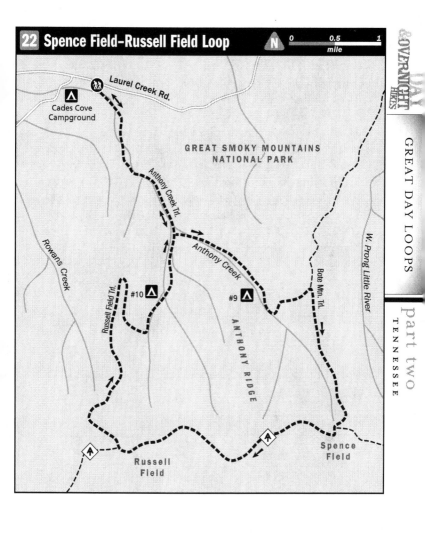

Laurel Creek Rd.

Cades Cove
Campground

GREAT SMOKY MOUNTAINS
NATIONAL PARK

Anthony Creek Trl.

Anthony Creek

Rowans Creek

W. Prong Little River

Russell Field Trl.

#10

#9

Bote Mtn. Trl.

ANTHONY RIDGE

Spence
Field

Russell
Field

Cove in Tennessee. It is an ideal spot to have a snack and rest before you turn west on the Appalachian Trail toward Russell Field. Before leaving Spence Field, the A.T. passes Eagle Creek Trail, where you'll find a backcountry shelter and a spring just a short way down at the meadow's southern edge.

Leave Spence Field on the Appalachian Trail and reenter the woods. Keep west through woodland, traveling gentle grades through the mountains. The A.T. descends, for the most part, to Russell Field and another trail shelter at mile 8.3. Just in front of the shelter is a trail junction and your departure from the A.T. Turn right on Russell Field Trail, passing the shelter spring before entering Russell Field. Today, the shrinking field is surrounded by forest but remains special despite the lack of views. You can't help but sense the serenity this highland meadow lends to those who pass through it.

Descend upon entering the forest, which eventually changes to pine-oak on easy-to-walk Leadbetter Ridge. At mile 10.1, leave Leadbetter Ridge and reenter the Anthony Creek watershed. Between the ridge and Leadbetter Ridge Backcountry Campsite 10, at mile 10.9, you'll traverse an old-growth forest with giant tulip

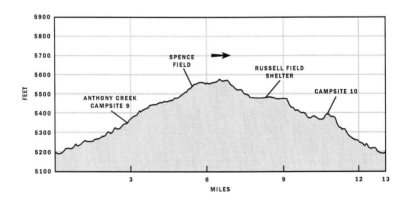

trees. At mile 11.7, you'll return to the intersection with Anthony Creek Trail. Retrace your steps down Anthony Creek to the Cades Cove picnic area.

DIRECTIONS: Just before the beginning of Cades Cove Loop Road, turn left toward the Cades Cove Campground, then turn left into the Cades Cove Picnic Area. Anthony Creek Trail will be on your right, at the rear of the picnic area. After finding the trailhead, return toward the campground and park your car in the lot beside the ranger station.

GPS Trailhead Coordinates	22 SPENCE FIELD— RUSSELL FIELD LOOP
Latitude:	N35° 35' 49.6"
Longitude:	W83° 45' 57.4"
UTM Zone (WGS 84):	17S
Easting:	0249400
Northing:	3942600

23 Baskins Creek Loop

SCENERY: ☆ ☆ ☆ ☆	DISTANCE: *5.8 miles*
DIFFICULTY: ☆ ☆ ☆	HIKING TIME: *3 hours*
TRAIL CONDITIONS: ☆ ☆ ☆ ☆	OUTSTANDING FEATURES: *Baskins Creek*
SOLITUDE: ☆ ☆	*Falls, ridgelines, pioneer cemetery*
CHILDREN: ☆ ☆ ☆ ☆	

This loop, very near Gatlinburg, travels hilly terrain past Baskins Creek Falls and some pioneer history before ending on the same road on which it started. Join Roaring Fork Motor Nature Trail for a bit, then take Trillium Gap Trail to complete your circuit.

🏃🏃 The area around Gatlinburg was heavily settled in prepark days, leading you to think that the terrain was more settlementfriendly than other parts of the park. In fact, however, its numerous hills and small, tight valleys challenged those who lived there.

Finding Baskins Creek Trail can be a challenge. It is best accessed where it crosses Roaring Fork Motor Nature Trail, 0.2 miles beyond the motor nature trail's beginning. Roaring Fork Motor Nature Trail is closed in winter, so during the cold time you will have to hike 0.2 miles from Cherokee Orchard to access the path. From the road, head left, as the hillier-than-you-think path innocently meanders through second-growth woodland before turning uphill onto an unnamed ridge spurring off Piney Mountain, a shoulder of Mount LeConte. Predictably, the woods turn piney here. Cruise along this attractive ridgeline before steeply descending to reach Falls Branch, a tributary of Baskins Creek. Step over the stream at 1 mile, and head downstream, soon passing a rock overhang on the right. This overhang would come in handy during a summer thunderstorm.

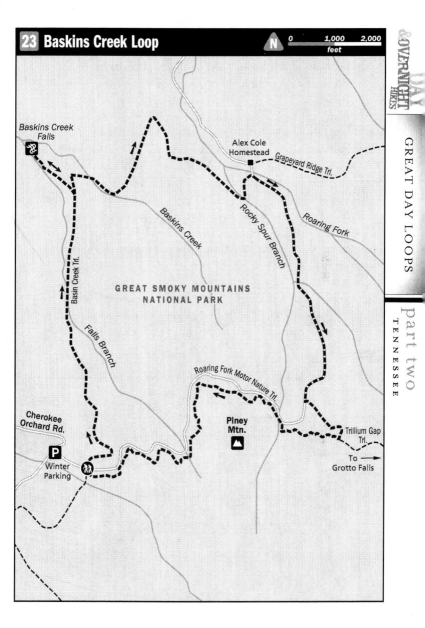

N

0   1,000   2,000
feet

Baskins Creek Falls

Alex Cole Homestead

Grapeyard Ridge Trl.

Rocky Spur Branch

Roaring Fork

Baskins Creek

Basin Creek Trl.

GREAT SMOKY MOUNTAINS NATIONAL PARK

Falls Branch

Roaring Fork Motor Nature Trl.

Piney Mtn.

Cherokee Orchard Rd.

P
Winter Parking

Trillium Gap Trl.

To →
Grotto Falls

Just as the hollow of Falls Branch becomes suffocatingly tight, it widens and reveals a sea of rhododendron below, where Falls Branch crashes downstream, seeking its level. Falls Branch is obscured by the rhododendron, but its descent fills the hollow with watery sounds. The path slips across a small flat to meet a spur trail leading left. This path travels a quarter mile uphill to Baskin Cemetery, a small pioneer internment. Baskins Creek Trail continues downstream to meet another spur trail at 1.3 miles. This is the path to Baskins Creek Falls. Waterfall enthusiasts will first trace the quarter-mile spur trail past a pioneer homesite, complete with broken-down chimney, and head down a muddy track. The flat where the homesite stands closes in, and the waterfall trail drops steeply to Baskins Creek Falls. You will likely be enjoying this cataract by yourself, while others throng to nearby Rainbow Falls and Grotto Falls.

Backtrack to the main trail, which curves uphill and over a ridge then drops to Baskins Creek. Step over the stream and you'll find an old wagon road that travels along Baskins Creek. Follow the main track up Baskins Creek, tunneling through rhododendron.

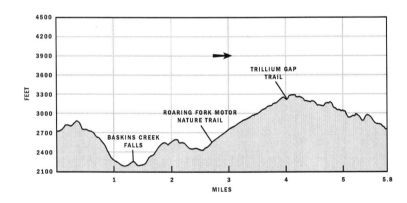

The hollow opens to a final homesite, the highest one on Baskins Creek, before turning up a dry drainage.

The subsequent 500-foot climb to the ridge dividing Baskins Creek from Rocky Spur Branch is steep. The trail levels out a bit on the ridgeline where chestnut oaks thrive, then descends to cross Rocky Spur Branch. Bales Cemetery is just beyond Rocky Spur Branch, on your right behind a fence. Most of the markers are vertical rock slabs without inscriptions, a simple memorial from a simpler time.

The path becomes gravel just before reaching Roaring Fork Motor Nature Trail at 2.7 miles. The Alex Cole homestead is just down the road and across Roaring Fork. Now, turn right, heading 1.2 miles up Roaring Fork Motor Nature Trail, then pick up the well-used connector path leading to the Trillium Gap Trail amid dying hemlocks to soon reach the actual Trillium Gap Trail. If you want to extend your loop, take a left to reach Grotto Falls, 1.1 miles distant. The main loop veers right on Trillium Gap Trail. This lesser used, nearly level path follows an old mountain roadbed crossing small creeks coming off the side of Mount LeConte. Doghobble, ferns, and rhododendron border the path as it passes above the parking area for Grotto Falls. Quartz outcrops brighten the woods. Watch for occasional big trees. The trail begins a downgrade before it reaches a trail junction near an incredibly gnarled oak tree. It is but a few feet to the right to reach Roaring Fork Road and the end of your loop at 5.8 miles.

DIRECTIONS: From the Sugarlands Visitor Center, take
US 441 north into Gatlinburg and on to traffic light number 8,
Airport Road. Turn right on Airport Road and drive 0.6 miles,
then continue, now on Cherokee Orchard Road, to enter the park.
At 4 miles, you'll reach Roaring Fork Motor Nature Trail. Keep
right here. At 0.2 miles you'll reach Baskins Creek Trail, on your
left. There is parking just beyond that.

GPS Trailhead Coordinates   23 BASKINS CREEK LOOP
              Latitude: N35° 40' 39.9"
             Longitude: W83° 28' 42.7"
    UTM Zone (WGS 84):   17S
               Easting: 0275690
              Northing: 3950810

24 Cucumber Gap Loop

SCENERY: ✿ ✿ ✿	DISTANCE: *5.3 miles*
DIFFICULTY: ✿ ✿	HIKING TIME: *3 hours*
TRAIL CONDITIONS: ✿ ✿ ✿ ✿ ✿	OUTSTANDING FEATURES: *River*
SOLITUDE: ✿ ✿ ✿	*environment, swimming potential*
CHILDREN: ✿ ✿ ✿ ✿	

This is a great hike for those who want more of a woodland stroll than a lung-busting mountain climb. Head out from Elkmont and cruise up the ultra-attractive Little River Valley, where the watercourse tumbles over huge boulders, forming large, clear pools that invite you to take a dip in the cool mountain stream. Leave Little River for an old railroad grade that gently climbs to a gap then descends to Jakes Creek Valley, from where you return to Elkmont.

🚶🚶 Start your hike on Little River Trail, which was moved in the mid-1990s after a flood washed out stretches of the upper section of the old road. Traverse the former Elkmont summer home community on a crumbling asphalt path. The trail soon turns to gravel. The sparkling Little River lies off to the left, always trying to lure you to its banks with attractive shoals, pools, and big rocks ideal for sunning.

At mile 1, pass the old parking area—here the path narrows. A bluff pinches the trail to the river in places. In other spots, Little River is only audible, not visible. At mile 2, the waterfall at Huskey Branch flows beneath a bridge into a large pool below. Look into the pool for the trout that lurk in its waters. Walk a bit farther to reach a trail junction at mile 2.3. Turn right here, on Cucumber Gap Trail, then ascend an old railroad grade, crossing Huskey Branch at mile 3.2. From the trail you will see numerous muscadine vines. There are more vines growing among the trees here than in any other part of the park.

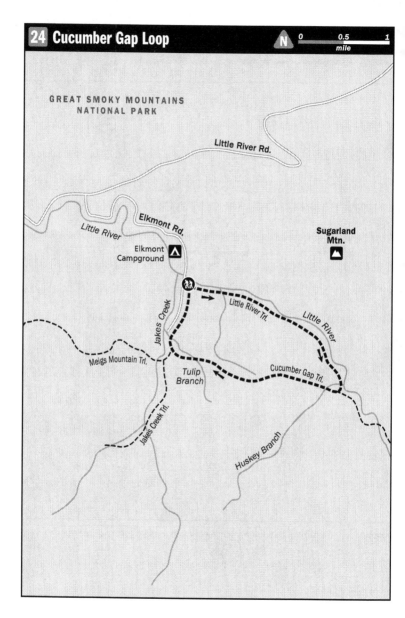

N

0   0.5   1
mile

GREAT SMOKY MOUNTAINS
NATIONAL PARK

Little River Rd.

Elkmont Rd.

Little River

Sugarland
Mtn.

Elkmont
Campground

Jakes Creek

Little River Trl.

Little River

Meigs Mountain Trl.

Tulip
Branch

Cucumber Gap Trl.

Jakes Creek Trl.

Huskey Branch

The path keeps rising along Huskey Branch's small feeder streams. Occasionally, there are impressive views through the trees to the right. The path passes just above Cucumber Gap, which was named for the cucumber tree—itself named for its green fruit, which resembles a mini cucumber. You can find these fruits trailside in September. Pass some fairly large beech and fading hemlock trees before descending to cross Tulip Branch at mile 4.4. Come to the wide Jakes Creek Trail at mile 4.6. Turn right here and descend to a pole gate at mile 4.9. Enter the former Elkmont summer home community and continue downhill on a crumbling asphalt path to a split in the road at mile 5.2. Turn right here and you'll soon reach Little River Trail, completing your loop at mile 5.3.

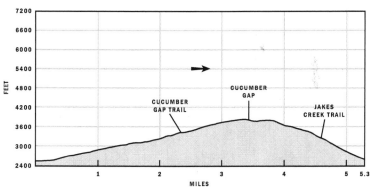

DIRECTIONS: Drive 4.9 miles from Sugarland Visitor Center before turning left into Elkmont. Follow the paved road 1.3 miles to the Elkmont Campground. Turn left just before the campground check-in station, and follow the road a short distance to a dead end. Little River Trail starts at the end of the gated road.

GPS Trailhead Coordinates	24 CUCUMBER GAP LOOP
Latitude:	N35° 39' 11.5"
Longitude:	W83° 34' 48.3"
UTM Zone (WGS 84):	17S
Easting:	0266410
Northing:	3948360

SCENERY: ✿ ✿ ✿ ✿	DISTANCE: *9.3 miles*
DIFFICULTY: ✿ ✿ ✿	HIKING TIME: *5 hours*
TRAIL CONDITIONS: ✿ ✿ ✿ ✿ ✿	OUTSTANDING FEATURES: *Big trees,*
SOLITUDE: ✿ ✿ ✿ ✿	*old pioneer homestead, Civil War gravesite*
CHILDREN: ✿ ✿ ✿	

Big trees are the stars of this loop, which starts in lovely Cataloochee Valley.
Of course, the numerous old-growth giants are complemented by other attractive
aspects of Smoky Mountain scenery. Add a visit to a pioneer homestead and you
end up with a great day in this national park. Start on Rough Fork Trail, tracing
a clear mountain stream. Stop by Woody Place, then enter the land of the giants,
where stately oak trees form a forest cathedral. Climb away from Rough Fork to meet
Caldwell Fork Trail. Descend past the "Big Poplars," in truth huge tulip trees,
then walk along Caldwell Fork Valley. Return over Big Fork Ridge to Cataloochee.
This loop has two climbs; neither is particularly long or difficult.

🚶 Start this loop on Rough Fork Trail. Pass around a pole
gate, with Rough Fork to the left. Cruise the wide, nearly level track
under a forest of maple, white pine, and yellow birch. The valley
soon narrows. Cross Rough Fork on a footbridge at 0.5 miles, then
twice more soon after. The path opens to a clearing and Woody Place
at 1 mile. This wood clapboard structure is worth a tour. A look
around reveals the differing ceiling heights, indicating that the structure was built in stages over time. There is also a springhouse nearby.

Rough Fork Trail continues to enter an old-growth woodland
of hemlock and northern red oak. Cross Hurricane Branch on a
long footbridge and come to Big Hemlock Campsite 40, an appropriately named backcountry campsite. A trail leads to the right to
access the actual camping area. The path, which has been nearly
level to this point, now climbs away from Big Hemlock toward Little

N

| 0 | 0.5 | 1 |

mile

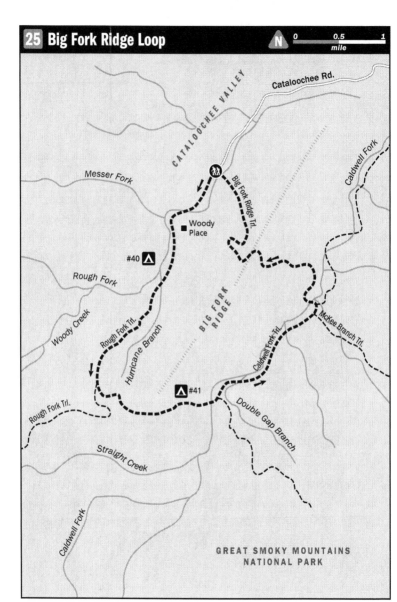

CATALOOCHEE VALLEY

Cataloochee Rd.

Messer Fork

Caldwell Fork

Big Fork Ridge Trl.

Woody Place

#40

Rough Fork

BIG FORK RIDGE

Woody Creek

Rough Fork Trl.

Hurricane Branch

McKee Branch Trl.

Caldwell Fork Trl.

#41

Rough Fork Trl.

Double Gap Branch

Straight Creek

Caldwell Fork

GREAT SMOKY MOUNTAINS
NATIONAL PARK

Ridge. Big tulip trees grow trailside. There are occasional views of Big Fork Ridge to the left. Top out on Little Ridge just before intersecting Caldwell Fork Trail at mile 3.

Turn left here on Caldwell Fork Trail and descend through more big trees into Caldwell Fork Valley. At mile 4.1, come to the side trail accessing the behemoth tulip trees, once mistakenly dubbed the "Big Poplars." These trees are huge and take several pairs of outstretched arms to encircle. Soon you pass through a former clearing and then reach Caldwell Fork Backcountry Campsite 41 and Hemphill Bald Trail, at mile 4.8. Keep descending along Caldwell Fork Valley; you'll reach a side trail leading to the right where there is a gravesite at mile 5.9. Further up this trail are the graves of two soldiers killed late in the Civil War. Meet McKee Branch Trail not far beyond the gravesite spur. Continue along Caldwell Fork Trail, which can be muddy in places, just a short distance farther to meet Big Fork Ridge Trail at mile 6.2.

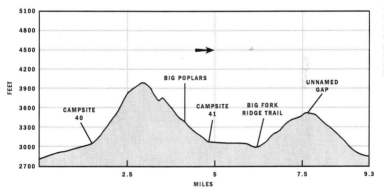

Make a dry crossing via a footbridge over Caldwell Fork on Big Fork Ridge Trail, and begin to wind up Big Fork Ridge, reaching a gap at mile 7.6. Descend into Rough Fork Valley. Here you reach a cove and a pioneer homesite, as evidenced by fields being reclaimed by forest. Cross Rough Fork on a footbridge to complete your loop at mile 9.3.

DIRECTIONS: From exit 20 on Interstate 40, head south a short distance on US 276. Turn right onto Cove Creek Road, which you will follow nearly 6 miles to enter the park. Two miles beyond the park boundary, turn left onto Cataloochee Road. Follow it to the dead end at Rough Fork Trail, which is at the end of the parking area.

GPS Trailhead Coordinates	25 BIG FORK RIDGE LOOP
Latitude:	N35° 37' 3.1"
Longitude:	W83° 7' 11.7"
UTM Zone (WGS 84):	17S
Easting:	0308000
Northing:	3943380

SCENERY: ☆ ☆ ☆ ☆ ☆	DISTANCE: 7.4 miles
DIFFICULTY: ☆ ☆ ☆	HIKING TIME: 3.25 hours
TRAIL CONDITIONS: ☆ ☆ ☆ ☆	OUTSTANDING FEATURES: Old homesites,
SOLITUDE: ☆ ☆ ☆ ☆	huge imperiled hemlocks, white pines, tulip trees
CHILDREN: ☆ ☆ ☆	

A footlog crossing is an appropriate beginning for this hike; you'll be quite familiar with them before this loop is over. But first, enjoy the beauty of huge trees, old homesites, and mountain streams on this fulfilling hike, whose trail name was the nickname of the man who owned the land, one Robert "Boogerman" Palmer. There is quite a bit of up and down, and the trail makers, while using old roads, make a few twists and turns to take you by the biggest trees in the area.

🚶🚶 Cross Cataloochee Creek on a footbridge and enter a stand of white pines. Where the trail splits, stay right and climb a narrow edge along Caldwell Fork. Descend, and you'll soon come to the north end of Boogerman Loop Trail, at mile 0.8. Turn left, crossing Caldwell Fork on a footbridge and entering an area of old-growth trees. Leave the cove and climb along a dry ridge before passing through a gap. White pines dominate the slope down to Boogerman's homestead at mile 2.8.

Hike away from the homestead and wind through a series of coves, where the trail intentionally nears many old tulip trees. If you look carefully, you'll notice that the tops have been sheared off most of these giants—the result of hundreds of years of rough living in the Smokies. At the last gap, the trail drops straight down and doubles as a streambed in wet weather. At mile 3.8 of your loop, the trail veers right, along Snake Branch and around a rock wall, then fords the small stream. Clearings, old fences, and piles of stone are other indicators of homesites along this creek.

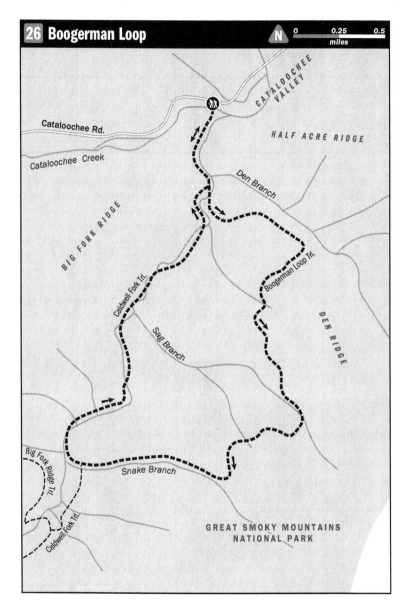

N

0   0.25   0.5
              miles

CATALOOCHEE VALLEY

Cataloochee Rd.

HALF ACRE RIDGE

Cataloochee Creek

Den Branch

BIG FORK RIDGE

Caldwell Fork Trl.

Boogerman Loop Trl.

Sag Branch

DEN RIDGE

Big Fork Ridge Trl.

Snake Branch

Caldwell Fork Trl.

GREAT SMOKY MOUNTAINS
NATIONAL PARK

More white pines signal your arrival at Caldwell Fork Trail junction at mile 4.6. Turn right and head down into this picturesque valley. Cross Snake Branch on a footlog and you'll soon start the nine footbridge crossings of Caldwell Fork amid the towering yet threatened hemlocks. Caldwell Fork Trail can be muddy and confusing; at stream crossings, the trail frequently splits. Hikers use footbridges, and horses ford the creek. Always take the trail headed for higher, drier ground.

These footbridges are a way to appreciate, without getting wet, the normally crystal-clear creek as you descend the valley, with its alternating deep pools and clamoring falls and riffles. At mile 6.6, come again to the northern junction of Boogerman Loop Trail. Continue down Caldwell Fork Trail, again passing the needle-carpeted area of white pines. The crossing of Cataloochee Creek on a footbridge at mile 7.4 signals completion of the loop.

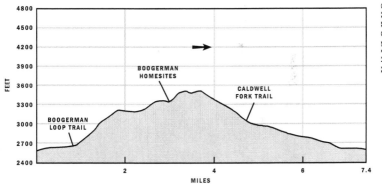

DIRECTIONS: Leave Iinterstate40 at exit 20 and drive west on NC 276, following it a short distance. Turn right onto Cove Creek Road, which you follow for nearly 6 miles to the park. Two miles beyond the park boundary, turn left onto the paved Cataloochee Road. Follow that 3.1 miles. Caldwell Fork Trail and its footbridge over Cataloochee Creek will be on your left.

GPS Trailhead Coordinates	26 BOOGERMAN LOOP
Latitude:	N35° 37' 53.0"
Longitude:	W83° 5' 16.3"
UTM Zone (WGS 84):	17S
Easting:	0310938
Northing:	3944887

27 Hyatt Ridge Loop

SCENERY: ✿ ✿ ✿ ✿	DISTANCE: *7.8 miles*
DIFFICULTY: ✿ ✿ ✿	HIKING TIME: *4.25 hours*
TRAIL CONDITIONS: ✿ ✿ ✿ ✿	OUTSTANDING FEATURES: *Isolation,*
SOLITUDE: ✿ ✿ ✿ ✿ ✿	*old-growth forest*
CHILDREN: ✿ ✿ ✿	

This loop hike takes you away from Straight Fork Road into the seldom-visited high country on Hyatt Ridge. Take the side trail to McGhee Spring Backcountry Campsite for lunch (this adds 1.8 miles to the hike), then return via Beech Gap Trail to Straight Fork. A short walk along the lightly used Straight Fork Road will complete your loop.

Start your trip on Hyatt Ridge Trail, beyond the gate on an old railroad grade, crossing Hyatt Creek at mile 0.7. Continue to ascend steeply through second-growth forest up the side of Hyatt Ridge. Come to Low Gap and a trail junction atop Hyatt Ridge (elevation 4,400 feet) at mile 1.9. Straight ahead is Enloe Creek Trail. Many spruce grow on this ridge.

Turn right, remaining on Hyatt Ridge Trail. Climb out of the gap for another 0.5 miles and come to an area of old-growth forest. Veer left, then make a sharp right turn to climb northeastward on Hyatt Bald, now wooded with a grassy understory, a reminder of its former state.

At mile 3.6, you come to another trail junction. This 0.9-mile trail leads to McGhee Spring Backcountry Campsite 44. At an elevation of 5,040 feet, this makes an excellent lunch spot beside a perennial spring in a mountain glade. To continue Hyatt Ridge Loop, turn right on Beech Gap Trail (once known as Hyatt Bald Trail). Sections of this trail feature tall, waving grasses beneath trees.

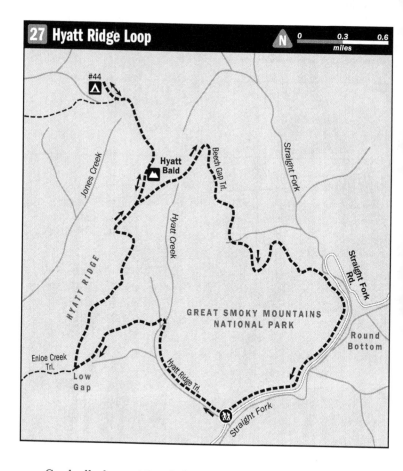

Gradually descend Beech Gap Trail, maintaining a north-eastward course. At mile 4.4, in a grassy gap, make a switchback to the right, leaving the ridgetop. Wind your way southward, passing the upper reaches of Grass Branch at mile 5.4. Soon the waters of

Straight Fork gurgle in the distance as the trail skirts more small branches to arrive at Straight Fork Road, at mile 6.5.

Turn right on Straight Fork Road, following its namesake stream down into Big Cove and Cherokee Reservation territory. This lightly used road actually makes for pleasant walking. You may encounter the occasional fisherman along the stream. Arrive at the Hyatt Ridge trailhead on your right at mile 7.8 to complete the loop.

DIRECTIONS: From the Oconaluftee Visitor Center, drive 1 mile south to Big Cove Road. Turn left, following it 10.4 miles through the Cherokee Reservation to the park boundary. Drive 2.5 miles beyond the boundary to the Hyatt Ridge trailhead, on your left.

GPS Trailhead Coordinates	27 HYATT RIDGE LOOP
Latitude:	N35° 36' 29.7"
Longitude:	W83° 13' 25.9"
UTM Zone (WGS 84):	17S
Easting:	0298560
Northing:	3942590

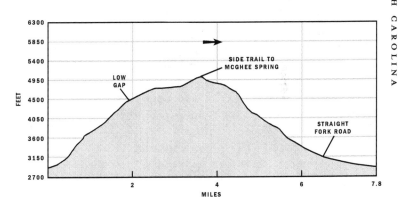

28 Smokemont Loop

SCENERY: ✿ ✿ ✿ ✿	DISTANCE: 5.4 miles
DIFFICULTY: ✿ ✿	HIKING TIME: 2.75 hours
TRAIL CONDITIONS: ✿ ✿ ✿ ✿ ✿	OUTSTANDING FEATURES: Good family day
SOLITUDE: ✿ ✿ ✿	hike through history and woods
CHILDREN: ✿ ✿ ✿ ✿	

This loop hike leads away from the popular Smokemont Campground along Bradley Fork, then upward along the southern reaches of Richland Mountain. The trail winds back down near the Oconaluftee River and past Bradley Cemetery, returning to the Smokemont campground.

🚶🚶 Start your loop hike on Bradley Fork Trail, at the rear of the Smokemont Campground. Pass an outbuilding, then a side road on your right leading to the water supply for the campground at mile 0.3. Open areas with thin forest cover indicate former homesites along the trail. At mile 1, cross a wide wooden bridge over Chasteen Creek, then come to the Chasteen Creek Trail junction. Press forward through the junction to reach the Smokemont Loop Trail junction at mile 1.6.

Turn left on Smokemont Loop Trail, crossing Bradley Fork on a long footbridge, then crossing a smaller branch on another footbridge. The narrow trail immediately switchbacks right, then left, swings around a knob on the way up Richland Mountain, and reaches the crest at mile 2.7. The white noise of the Oconaluftee River accompanies you on your southward journey along Richland Mountain.

The trail reaches its high point, nearly 3,500 feet, at mile 3.4. A couple of downed logs invite a rest here. The trail then begins to wind down the slope of Richland Mountain, alternately flanked by

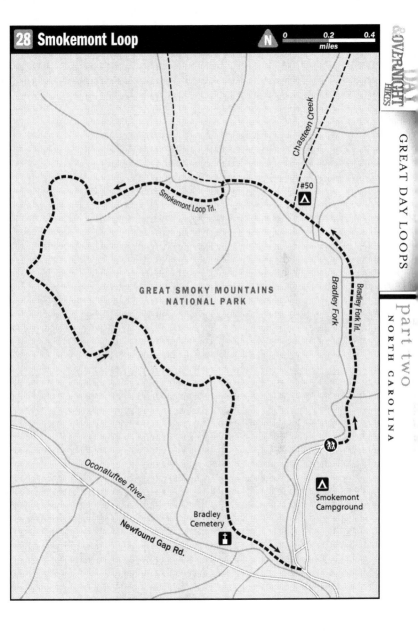

0   0.2   0.4
miles

Chasteen Creek

Smokemont Loop Trl.

#50

Bradley Fork

Bradley Fork Trl.

GREAT SMOKY MOUNTAINS
NATIONAL PARK

Oconaluftee River

Newfound Gap Rd.

Bradley Cemetery

Smokemont Campground

open woods and thick rhododendron. At mile 5, Bradley Cemetery appears on your right, farther along the trail. Continue down to a jeep road that used to loop through a now closed section of the Smokemont Campground, and turn right to reach a side trail to the cemetery, climbing a small hill. Worn stones marking the graves of settlers whose names are lost to time stand beside gravestones with names still legible.

Return to the jeep road and follow it over Bradley Fork on an old stone bridge back to the Smokemont Campground at mile 5.4, completing your loop. The Bradley Fork trailhead is to your left at the rear of the campground.

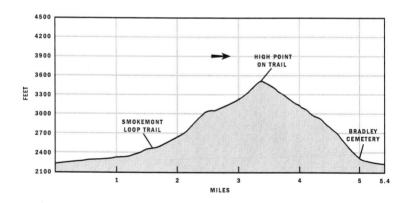

DIRECTIONS: From the Oconaluftee Visitor Center, drive 3.2 miles north on Newfound Gap Road. Turn right into the Smokemont Campground on a bridge over the Oconaluftee River. Veer left and pass the campground check-in station. Bradley Fork Trail starts at the gated jeep road at the right rear of the campground as you enter.

GPS Trailhead Coordinates	28 SMOKEMONT LOOP
Latitude:	N35° 33' 43.2"
Longitude:	W83° 18' 42.5"
UTM Zone (WGS 84):	17S
Easting:	0290450
Northing:	3937650

29 Indian Creek Loop

SCENERY: ☆☆☆☆	DISTANCE: 12.4 miles
DIFFICULTY: ☆☆☆☆	HIKING TIME: 6.5 hours
TRAIL CONDITIONS: ☆☆☆☆	OUTSTANDING FEATURES: Indian Creek Falls,
SOLITUDE: ☆☆☆	quiet ridge
CHILDREN: ☆☆	

The biological diversity of the Smokies can be well appreciated on this trek, which follows lush Deep Creek to Indian Creek, then passes Indian Creek Falls to climb to Martins Gap and return via the quiet Sunkota Ridge Trail, with its drier forest, before taking you back to Deep Creek and its riverine habitat.

🏃 Start your hike on Deep Creek Trail at the end of Deep Creek Road just beyond Deep Creek Campground. Follow an old gravel road, crossing Deep Creek on a bridge en route to the junction with Indian Creek Trail at 0.7 miles. Turn right on Indian Creek Trail and you'll reach Indian Creek Falls at 0.8 miles. A spur path leads to the base of the falls. Continuing along Indian Creek, Stone Pile Gap Trail leaves right at 1.2 miles. Then, at mile 1.5, the Loop Trail heads up Sunkota Ridge to your left. Stay north on Indian Creek Trail.

A series of pioneer homesites appears along Indian Creek, between several bridged crossings. At 3.6 miles a gradual climb has led you to the Deeplow Gap Trail. Continue following the Indian Creek Trail to its end at mile 4.6, in a road turnaround near Estes Branch. Here starts Martins Gap Trail.

Keep hiking through the turnaround to join Martins Gap Trail. Span Indian Creek three times in a half mile on footbridges before switchbacking up the side of Sunkota Ridge to arrive at Martins Gap, at 6.4 miles. Martins Gap, a sag on Sunkota Ridge, has a four-way

134

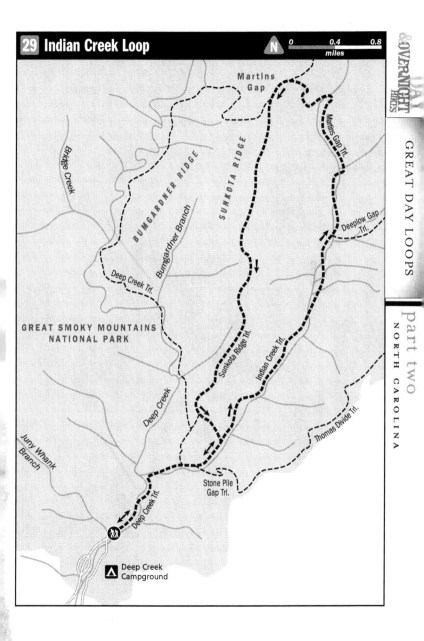

N

0   0.4   0.8
miles

Martins
Gap

Martins Gap Trl.

Deeplow Gap Trl.

BUMGARDNER RIDGE

SUNKOTA RIDGE

Bridge
Creek

Bumgardner Branch

Deep Creek Trl.

GREAT SMOKY MOUNTAINS
NATIONAL PARK

Deep Creek

Sunkota Ridge Trl.

Indian Creek Trl.

Thomas Divide Trl.

Juny Whank
Branch

Deep Creek Trl.

Stone Pile
Gap Trl.

Deep Creek Trl.

Deep Creek
Campground

trail intersection. Turn left on the serene Sunkota Ridge Trail. "Sunkota" is the pioneer spelling of the Indian word for "apple."

Climb out of the gap to the loop's high point at mile 7.2 and begin a slow descent, winding along the ridgetop and its flanks. Enjoy the forest cruise. At mile 10.2, Sunkota Ridge Trail ends at the Loop Trail. Turn right, as Loop Trail meets Deep Creek Trail at mile 10.7. Follow Deep Creek Trail downstream over three bridges to Indian Creek Trail at mile 11.7, then backtrack a half mile to the trailhead.

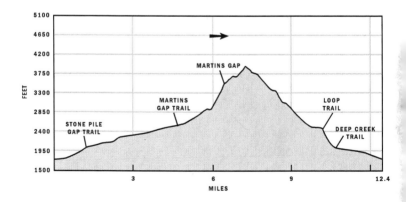

DIRECTIONS: From the Oconaluftee Visitor Center, take US 441 south to Cherokee. Turn right on US 19 to head toward Bryson City. Turn right at the Swain County Courthouse onto Everett Street and carefully follow the signs through town to Deep Creek Campground. Deep Creek Trail is behind the campground.

GPS Trailhead Coordinates	29 INDIAN CREEK LOOP
Latitude:	N35° 27' 34.6"
Longitude:	W83° 26' 18.6"
UTM Zone (WGS 84):	17S
Easting:	0278722
Northing:	3926527

30 Goldmine Loop

SCENERY: ✿ ✿ ✿ ✿	DISTANCE: *3.3 miles*
DIFFICULTY: ✿	HIKING TIME: *1.75 hours*
TRAIL CONDITIONS: ✿ ✿ ✿ ✿	OUTSTANDING FEATURES: *Fontana Lake,*
SOLITUDE: ✿ ✿ ✿ ✿ ✿	*Lakeview Tunnel, homesites*
CHILDREN: ✿ ✿ ✿ ✿ ✿	

This short loop hike traverses a seldom-visited area of the Smokies. Beginning at Lakeview Drive, you hike down to Fontana Lake. The trail moves away from the lake, passing several old homesites along the way, then returns to Lakeview Drive through Lakeview Tunnel. Several old roads and trails branch off Goldmine Loop Trail, so watch your direction.

🚶🚶 The loop hike starts near the parking area at the end of Lakeview Drive. With your back to the parking lot, begin your hike on Tunnel Bypass Trail, just across the road and to the left. Once on the trail, descend briefly through a rhododendron thicket and then climb up to a small gap at mile 0.3. An old trail below leads to the same gap. Proceed through the gap, skirting a knob to arrive at another gap and a trail junction on a modest ridge at mile 0.5.

Turn left on Goldmine Loop Trail and descend a ridge on the narrow path. You'll come to an old road that parallels Tunnel Branch; veer right. The forest is more closed-in here than on the ridgetop. The old road turns away from Tunnel Branch and comes to Fontana Lake at mile 1.3.

The trail will intersect another road that swings around and over a tiny creek, then passes over Hyatt Branch via stone culverts. At mile 1.7, you'll come to the side trail leading to Goldmine Branch Backcountry Campsite 67. The campsite is located in an open homesite a few hundred yards up the side trail.

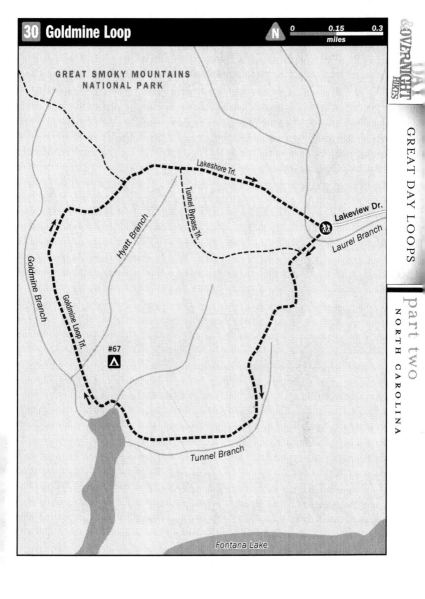

N

0   0.15   0.3
miles

GREAT SMOKY MOUNTAINS
NATIONAL PARK

Lakeshore Trl.

Lakeview Dr.

Laurel Branch

Tunnel Bypass Trl.

Hyatt Branch

Goldmine Branch

Goldmine Loop Trl.

#67

Tunnel Branch

Fontana Lake

Goldmine Loop Trail recrosses Goldmine Branch on a culvert then becomes muddy. Beyond the muddy area, the trail briefly leaves the road and skirts the right side of a homesite. Goldmine Loop Trail rejoins the old road to reach a second homesite at mile 2.2.

A stone chimney stands near the trail. Swing past the homesite through a rhododendron tunnel to emerge at the top of the hollow. The road continues straight, but the trail makes a sharp right alongside a ridge to a saddle. Next, the path veers left for a short but steep climb to intersect Lakeshore Trail at mile 2.6.

Turn right on Lakeshore Trail and, within a scant 100 yards, you'll come to a junction with Tunnel Bypass Trail. Pass through the junction to reach Lakeview Tunnel at mile 2.9. Walk the 0.2-mile-long tunnel and emerge near Lakeview Drive to complete your 3.3-mile loop.

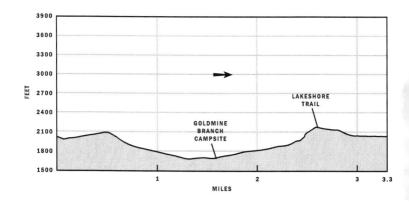

DIRECTIONS: From the Oconaluftee Visitor Center, head south on Newfound Gap Road 3.2 miles to US 19 in Cherokee, North Carolina. Turn right on US 19 and follow it 10 miles to Bryson City, North Carolina. Once in Bryson City, turn right at the courthouse and continue straight on Everett Street, which soon becomes Lakeview Drive. The parking area is 7.9 miles from the courthouse in Bryson City, at the end of Lakeview Drive.

GPS Trailhead Coordinates	30 GOLDMINE LOOP
Latitude:	N35° 27' 29.5"
Longitude:	W83° 32' 13.3"
UTM Zone (WGS 84):	17S
Easting:	0269730
Northing:	3926630

31 Twentymile Loop

SCENERY: ☆ ☆ ☆ ☆	DISTANCE: *7.4 miles*
DIFFICULTY: ☆ ☆	HIKING TIME: *3.75 hours*
TRAIL CONDITIONS: ☆ ☆ ☆	OUTSTANDING FEATURES: *waterfall,*
SOLITUDE: ☆ ☆ ☆ ☆ ☆	*mountain streams, deep woods*
CHILDREN: ☆ ☆ ☆ ☆	

This streamside loop hike never gets too far from the sound of falling water, one of the key ingredients of Smokies ambiance. This is one of the most rewarding out-of-the-way trips in the park. The hike travels along Twentymile Creek then veers left on Wolf Ridge Trail, with Moore Spring Branch, a fine trout stream, as your noisy companion. Turn east on Twentymile Loop Trail to hike into deep woods, over Long Hungry Ridge, and down to Twentymile Trail. Follow Twentymile Creek as it cascades down toward Cheoah Lake.

Start your loop on Twentymile Trail, following it to mile 0.6, then hike over the bridged crossing of Moore Spring Branch to the Wolf Ridge Trail junction. Turn left on Wolf Ridge Trail to cross Moore Spring Branch on footlogs three times in the first half mile. Cross Moore Spring Branch without the benefit of footlogs at mile 1.3 and 1.5.

At mile 1.6, the Twentymile Loop Trail junction, turn right. Twentymile Loop Trail heads east, fording Moore Spring Branch yet again, then ascends toward a gap. After some meandering up the side of Long Hungry Ridge, the trail passes through a sag in the ridge at mile 3.2, Hickory Nut Gap.

Twentymile Loop Trail soon slopes sharply down heavily wooded Long Hungry Ridge, an ideal place to pause and absorb the essence of a southern Appalachian forest. Ford Twentymile Creek at mile 4.2, then cross a level area before rising to Proctor Gap and a trail junction at mile 4.4.

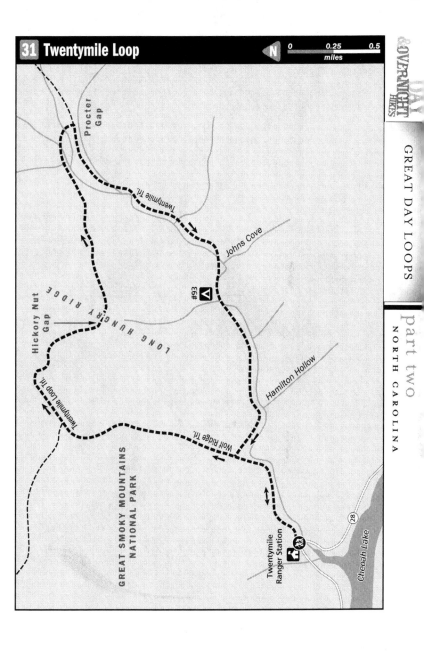

N

0   0.25   0.5
miles

Procter Gap

Twentymile Trl.

Johns Cove

#93

Hickory Nut Gap

LONG HUNGRY RIDGE

Twentymile Loop Trl.

Hamilton Hollow

Wolf Ridge Trl.

GREAT SMOKY MOUNTAINS
NATIONAL PARK

Twentymile
Ranger Station

28

Cheoah Lake

Turn right on Twentymile Trail, following its namesake, Twentymile Creek, downstream. Just after crossing a wide bridge, come to Twentymile Creek Backcountry Campsite 93, at mile 5.7. Cross two more bridges in quick succession to arrive at the side trail for Twentymile Cascades at mile 6.7. Take the side trail to view the waterfall that descends in stages. At mile 6.8, your previous turnoff, Wolf Ridge Trail joins the path from the right. Follow Twentymile Trail past the horse barn and back to the trailhead at mile 7.4.

DIRECTIONS: From Townsend, Tennessee, take U.S. 321 north to the Foothills Parkway. Follow Foothills Parkway west to U.S. 129 south into North Carolina. Turn left on NC 28. Follow NC 28 for 2.6 miles to Twentymile Ranger Station, on your left. Park beyond the ranger station and walk up to the gated road and begin your hike on the Twentymile Trail. From the courthouse in Bryson City, N.C., take U.S. 19 south for 5.4 miles to NC 28. Follow NC 28 thirty miles to Twentymile Ranger Stations, which will be on your right.

GPS Trailhead Coordinates   31 TWENTYMILE LOOP
Latitude: N35° 28' 9.9"
Longitude: W83° 52' 18.8"
UTM Zone (WGS 84):   17S
Easting: 0239350
Northing: 3928700

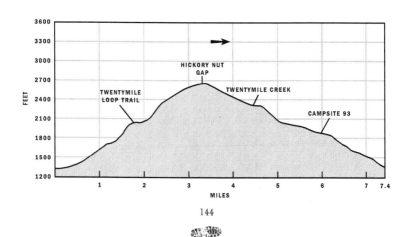

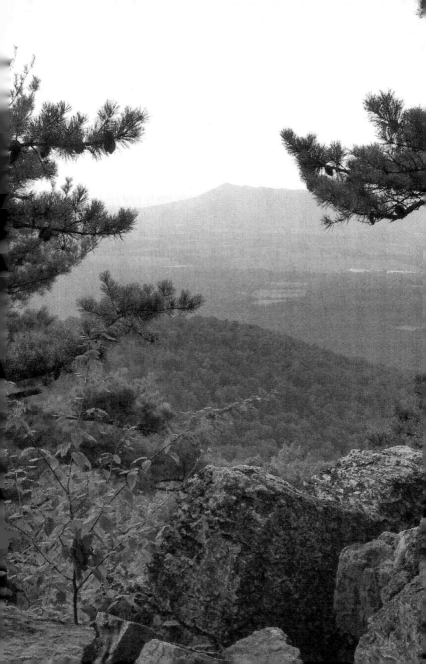

part three
GREAT OVERNIGHT LOOPS

3

The return
trip to the
AT will
get you
huffing and
puffing
while
thinking of
all the
people that
skipped
this
second view
as is
evidenced
by the
much less
used trail
tread

32 Gregory Bald Overnight Loop

SCENERY: ✿ ✿ ✿ ✿ ✿	DISTANCE (PER DAY): *4.1, 4.6, 7 miles*
DIFFICULTY: ✿ ✿ ✿	HIKING TIME (PER DAY): *2.5, 3, 4 hours*
TRAIL CONDITIONS: ✿ ✿ ✿ ✿	OUTSTANDING FEATURES: *good campsites,*
SOLITUDE: ✿ ✿ ✿ ✿	*high-country meadows*
CHILDREN: ✿ ✿	

This hike combines the best that the high and low country have to offer. First, you'll travel the Twentymile Trail past Twentymile Cascades to the Upper Flats streamside camp. Then an arduous climb tops out on Long Hungry Ridge and leads to Gregory Bald Trail, arriving at the most famous bald in southern Appalachia, with its staggering views and flower displays. Camp at Sheep Pen Gap, a high-country grassy glade between Gregory Bald and Parson Bald. Leave the grassy balds and complete your loop via the steep Wolf Ridge Trail.

🚶 Start your hike on the Twentymile Trail, following it to Wolf Ridge Trail junction at mile 0.6. Turn right, passing the side trail to Twentymile Cascades on your right at mile 0.7. Climb moderately, passing over Twentymile Creek on wide bridges at miles 1.4 and 1.6. Just beyond the second crossing is Twentymile Creek Backcountry Campsite 93. Cross another bridge behind the campsite. The trail climbs above the creek, then drops down and crosses Twentymile Creek twice more on bridges before coming to Proctor Gap at mile 3.

Stay on the old railroad bed to pick up Long Hungry Ridge Trail, crossing Proctor Creek at mile 3.1. Swing around the point of a ridge, then come alongside Twentymile Creek again. The rotting bridges on the side streams are remnants of the logging era, in which railroads were built to haul timber. These bridges are dangerous! Do not try to use them to cross the creek. At mile 4.1, come to Upper Flats Backcountry Campsite 92 (elevation 2,520 feet). This is your first night's destination. Upper Flats has several good tent sites.

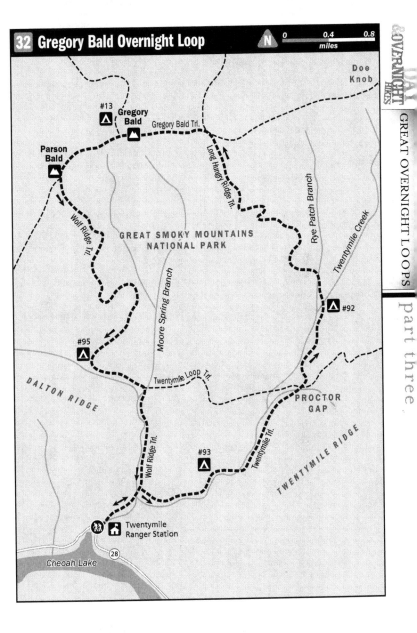

N

0   0.4   0.8
miles

Doe Knob

#13
Gregory Bald

Gregory Bald Trl.

Parson Bald

Long Hungry Ridge Trl.

Wolf Ridge Trl.

GREAT SMOKY MOUNTAINS
NATIONAL PARK

Rye Patch Branch

Twentymile Creek

Moore Spring Branch

#92

#95

Twentymile Loop Trl.

DALTON RIDGE

PROCTOR
GAP

Wolf Ridge Trl.

#93

Twentymile Trl.

TWENTYMILE RIDGE

Twentymile
Ranger Station

Cheoah Lake

28

Large rocks emerge from the ground, forming natural seats at the campsite.

Start day two by immediately crossing Twentymile Creek, then Rye Patch Branch. The once-moderate grade becomes steep as the trail crosses Rye Patch Branch at mile 4.6 of your loop hike before ascending the dry hillside. After a sharp right turn, you'll come to Rye Patch (elevation 4,500 feet) at mile 6.8. This formerly open area is rapidly growing over but still remains an ideal resting spot after you've made the climb to the crest of Long Hungry Ridge.

Now atop the ridge, the last 0.8 miles of Long Hungry Ridge Trail is easy, ending at the Gregory Bald Trail junction at mile 7.6. Turn left on Gregory Bald Trail and you'll soon come to Rich Gap and another trail junction at mile 7.7. If you are thirsty, turn left on the unmarked side trail and go 0.3 miles to Moore Spring, site of an old Appalachian Trail shelter. From Rich Gap, continue on Gregory Bald Trail and climb 0.6 miles to the grassy meadow of Gregory Bald at mile 8.3. The bald, maintained at 15 acres by the park service, offers a nearly 360-degree view. Flame azaleas bloom in June and blueberries follow.

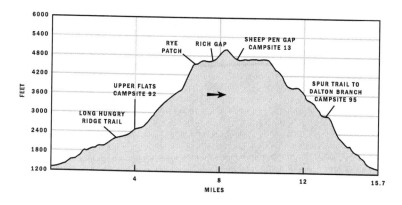

Reenter the woods on the western end of the bald and descend to the Wolf Ridge Trail junction and Sheep Pen Gap Backcountry Campsite 13 (elevation 4,560 feet), at mile 8.7. This is your second night's destination, a grassy glade of open, level woodland—one of the Smokies' finest backcountry campsites. Make sure and call to get a spot at this rationed campsite. You can find water at a spring 200 yards down Gregory Bald Trail, on your left. Sunset from atop Gregory Bald is a Smoky Mountain sight not to be missed.

Start day three by heading southwest on Wolf Ridge Trail through level grassy woodland. Come to Parson Bald at mile 9.5 of your loop hike. This bald, unlike Gregory Bald, is not maintained by the park service and is rapidly filling with trees and bushes, which limit views. But look over your left shoulder as you enter the clearing to view grassy Gregory Bald. Leave the bald and continue on a nearly level hike for another 0.8 miles, then begin an intermittent but steep descent down Wolf Ridge.

Swing right toward Dalton Branch, coming to the side trail leading to Dalton Branch Backcountry Campsite 95, at mile 13.1. Veer left beyond the campsite and pick up an old road that descends steeply to Twentymile Loop Trail junction at mile 14.1. Wolf Ridge Trail then crosses Moore Spring Branch at miles 14.2 and 14.4. In the next 0.7 miles, cross Moore Spring Branch three times on footlogs to arrive at the Twentymile Trail junction, at mile 15.1. Cross Moore Spring Branch one last time, just beyond the junction, and follow Twentymile Trail 0.6 miles to the trailhead, completing your loop.

DIRECTIONS: From Townsend, Tennessee, take US 321 north to Foothills Parkway. Follow Foothills Parkway west to US 129, then take US 129 south into North Carolina. Turn left on NC 28 and follow it 2.6 miles to Twentymile Ranger Station, on your left. Park beyond the ranger station and walk up to the gated road to begin your hike on Twentymile Trail. From the courthouse in Bryson City, North Carolina, take US 19 south 5.4 miles to NC 28. Drive 30 miles on NC 28 to reach Twentymile Ranger Station, on your right.

GPS Trailhead Coordinates	32 GREGORY BALD OVERNIGHT LOOP
Latitude:	N35° 28' 9.9"
Longitude:	W83° 52' 18.8"
UTM Zone (WGS 84):	17S
Easting:	0239350
Northing:	3928700

33 Little River Overnight Loop

SCENERY: ✿ ✿ ✿ ✿	DISTANCE (PER DAY): *6.1, 7.6, 5.8 miles*
DIFFICULTY: ✿ ✿ ✿	HIKING TIME (PER DAY): *3.25, 4, 3 hours*
TRAIL CONDITIONS: ✿ ✿ ✿ ✿	OUTSTANDING FEATURES: *Views, attractive*
SOLITUDE: ✿ ✿ ✿	*streams, multiple environments*
CHILDREN: ✿ ✿ ✿	

This overnight loop follows the Little River deep into the heart of the Smokies, where you will camp in the shadow of Clingmans Dome. Then you'll ascend Sugarland Mountain via Rough Creek Trail and camp in a boulder field at the little-used Medicine Branch Bluff campsite. This trip offers creekside and ridgeline camping with a fair amount of climbing in between.

🚶🚶 Start your camping trip on Little River Trail, tracing an old railroad grade. Pass the remains of the Elkmont vacation home enclave. The cascading Little River offers an ever-changing water show to your left. The stream crashes amid rocks only to gather in large pools that fall again in a white, frothy mix of water and air. At mile 2, Huskey Branch enters the Little River in a fall above the trail, which bridges the small creek. Cucumber Gap Trail enters from the west at mile 2.3.

Continue up the Little River, crossing it on a wide bridge just before the Huskey Gap Trail junction at mile 2.7. Stay on the east bank of the Little River, crossing several small feeder streams originating on Sugarland Mountain, and you will reach a wide flat near the confluence of Goshen Prong and the Little River, at mile 3.7. Goshen Prong Trail bears right; stay on Little River Trail to reach Rough Creek Backcountry Campsite 24, at mile 4.5.

Little River Trail becomes somewhat rockier as it passes the Rough Creek trail junction, just beyond the campsite. Look for the even spacing of old railroad ties. Continue on Little River Trail,

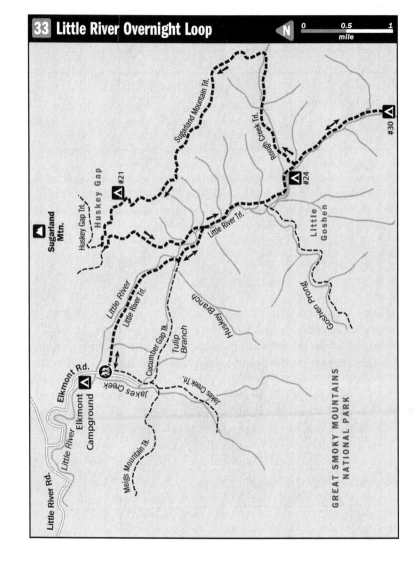

N

0   0.5   1
mile

Sugarland Mountain Trl.

Rough Creek Trl.

#21

Huskey Gap

Huskey Gap Trl.

#24

#30

Sugarland Mtn.

Little Goshen

Little River Trl.

Goshen Prong

Little River

Little River Trl.

Huskey Branch

Cucumber Gap Trl.

Tulip Branch

Jakes Creek Trl.

Little River Rd.

Elkmont Rd.

Little River

Elkmont Campground

Jakes Creek

Meigs Mountain Trl.

GREAT SMOKY MOUNTAINS
NATIONAL PARK

crossing Meigs Post Prong at mile 5.7, where the remains of an old railroad bridge lie about the creek bed.

Cross what's left of the Little River at mile 6.1, where another old railroad bridge is particularly evident, to arrive at Three Forks Backcountry Campsite 30. At elevation 3,400 feet, this former logging camp is your first night's destination. Native brook trout populate the high-country streams that border this grassy area on three sides.

Start day two by backtracking 1.6 miles down Little River Trail to meet Rough Creek Trail at mile 7.7. Turn right and begin climbing Rough Creek Trail, which also follows an old railroad bed, through second-growth forest. As you climb, notice the various remnants of railroad days. After crossing Rough Creek three times, the trail runs north to intersect Sugarland Mountain Trail on the narrow ridge at mile 10.5.

Turn left on Sugarland Mountain Trail. Meander along the ridgetop, staying near 4,500 feet in elevation for the next 1.7 miles, before descending around the southern side of a knob on Sugarland Mountain. After working past a point in the ridge, veer into the

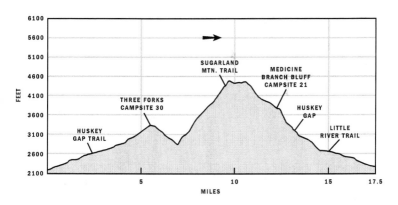

Big Medicine Branch hollow. Medicine Branch Bluff Backcountry Campsite 21, is in a boulder field at mile 13.7. This site is your second night's destination. This lightly used site, at 3,780 feet, is on a fair slope, but a few flat tent sites hide among the boulders. Water can be obtained from the small stream flowing at the base of the hollow.

To begin day three, continue northwest on Sugarland Mountain Trail. At mile 14.7 of the loop is a junction with Huskey Gap Trail. Turn left on Huskey Gap Trail, an old prepark crossroads, descending past the drainages of Big Medicine Branch and Phoebe Branch to enter a wide, flat area near the Little River. Arrive at Little River Trail just after crossing Sugar Orchard Branch at mile 16.8.

Head down Little River Trail, once again passing the Cucumber Gap Trail at mile 17.2. Walk along the west bank of the river to arrive at the trailhead, and the end of your loop, at mile 18.5.

DIRECTIONS: Drive 4.9 miles from Sugarland Visitor Center, then turn left into Elkmont. Follow the paved road 1.3 miles to the Elkmont Campground. Turn left just before the campground check-in station and follow the road a short distance to a dead end. Little River Trail starts at the end of the gated road.

GPS Trailhead Coordinates	33 LITTLE RIVER OVERNIGHT LOOP
Latitude:	N35° 39' 11.5"
Longitude:	W83° 34' 48.3"
UTM Zone (WGS 84):	17S
Easting:	0266410
Northing:	3948360

SCENERY: ✿ ✿ ✿ ✿ ✿	DISTANCE (PER DAY): 6.7, 5.5, 12.8 miles
DIFFICULTY: ✿ ✿ ✿ ✿	HIKING TIME (PER DAY): 4, 2.75, 7.75
TRAIL CONDITIONS: ✿ ✿ ✿ ✿	OUTSTANDING FEATURES: Views, attractive
SOLITUDE: ✿ ✿ ✿	streams, multiple environments
CHILDREN: ✿	

This loop starts at the highest trailhead in the park, taking the Appalachian Trail past myriad views of the park and beyond. It then drops into Tennessee, where you leave the high-country spruce–fir forest for a streamside campsite in rich woodland that has everywhere-you-look beauty. Remain in Little River Valley for a lovely watershed walk, to spend your second night beneath Clingmans Dome at Three Forks. Get a good night's sleep here because your final day sees a long and strenuous climb back to the high country via Sugarland Mountain Trail, with more good views along the way. Finally, intersect the Appalachian Trail to undulate over Mount Collins and Clingmans Dome. Make a final stop at the observation tower atop the dome before completing your loop.

Start your loop hike at the Clingmans Dome parking area, leaving on Forney Ridge Trail through a spruce–fir forest. At 0.1 mile, veer right on Clingmans Dome Bypass Trail. After a moderate half-mile climb, intersect the Appalachian Trail near Mount Buckley, elevation 6,500 feet. Continue west on the A.T., dropping through an area that bears fire scars. This section of trail offers impressive views, thanks to the low-lying recovering vegetation. Drop into a saddle, then ascend again briefly, topping a rock outcrop that makes a wonderful bench for gazing across North Carolina.

Enter the spruce–fir forest again, moving downward all the while. It is nearly always wet and cool here, pungent with the aroma of rich earth and growing and decaying vegetation. After a brief level section, come to Goshen Prong Trail at mile 2.7. Turn right here

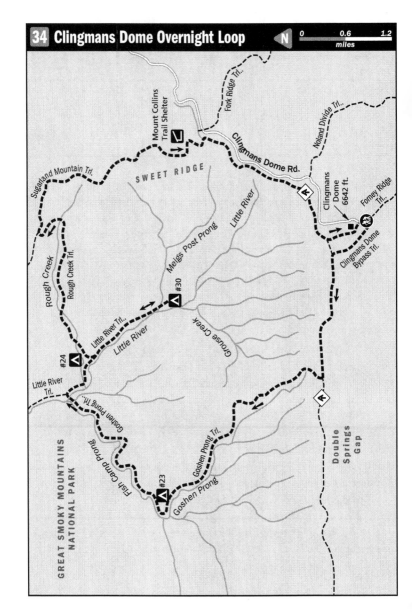

N

0   0.6   1.2
          miles

Fork Ridge Trl.

Mount Collins Trail Shelter

Noland Divide Trl.

Clingmans Dome Rd.

Suganland Mountain Trl.

SWEET RIDGE

Clingmans Dome 6642 ft.

Forney Ridge Trl.

Little River

Little River

Rough Creek

Rough Creek Trl.

Meigs Post Prong

Clingmans Dome Bypass Trl.

△ #30

Little River Trl.

Little River

Grouse Creek

#24 △

Little River Trl.

Goshen Prong Trl.

Double Springs Gap

Fish Camp Prong

Goshen Prong Trl.

△ #23

Goshen Prong

GREAT SMOKY MOUNTAINS NATIONAL PARK

and descend on a rocky path, entering Tennessee. Spruce and yellow birch dominate the woodland. There are good views of the Volunteer State. Pass a spring branch at mile 3. Rhododendron and Fraser fir line the path.

At mile 3.8, the trail swings right, passing a slope of moss-covered rocks. Goshen Prong becomes audible by mile 4.8. Keep descending into the Goshen Prong watershed, soon passing a curious, three-foot-high cave. Follow one of Goshen Prong's feeder streams, which forms a waterfall on a tilted rock face. Saddle alongside Goshen Prong to pick up an old railroad grade at mile 5.4. The descent continues. Watch the trail for pieces of coal that once fired the trains' engines. The path leaves the grade and is pinched between Goshen Prong on the left and a bluff on the right.

Enter a flat, and you will come to a trail sign at mile 6.6. Turn right here, still on Goshen Prong Trail, and reach the spur trail to Camp Rock Backcountry Campsite 23. The large camp, shaded by yellow birches, has many level sites; this is your first night's destination. Water can be obtained from Fish Camp Prong, just across the main path.

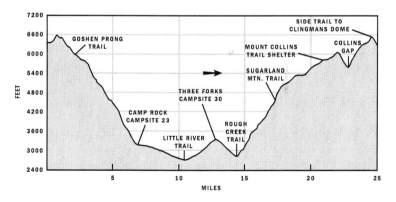

Start your second day by continuing down Goshen Prong Trail, immediately crossing Fish Camp Prong. Northern hardwoods tower over Fish Camp Prong's pools and cascades. Occasional streamside flats and rock bluffs add scenic variation. At mile 7.1 of your loop hike, pass the old, long-closed, Camp Rock campsite in an open flat to the left. Leave the railroad grade you have been following and climb away from the stream on a steep path before dropping back down to Fish Camp Prong.

You'll come to an old traffic circle at mile 9.1. Young trees are growing in the center of the circle. Continue down the widening valley to meet the Little River. An iron bridge spans the stream where a railroad bridge stood long ago. Continue straight, past the bridge, and you'll reach an intersection with Little River Trail at mile 9.9. Turn right here, and begin a moderate ascent on an old railroad grade, reaching Rough Creek Backcountry campsite 24 at mile 10.6. Continue and you'll soon pass Rough Creek Trail, which leaves left. Save this trail for tomorrow. Hiking forward on Little River Trail, you'll crossing Meigs Post Prong at mile 11.8, where signs of an old railroad bridge lie about the creek bed. Although you'll see evidence of camping here, this is not a legal camping area. Continue on to the real Three Forks campsite, which you'll reach after crossing what's left of the Little River at mile 12.2, where another old railroad bridge is evident. Here you arrive at Three Forks Backcountry Campsite 30, at 3,400 feet, once the site of a logging camp. This is your second night's destination, where you'll sleep in a grassy area surrounded by a birch forest, bounded on three sides by high-country streams. Be prepared for a long day tomorrow!

Start day three by backtracking 1.6 miles down Little River Trail to Rough Creek Trail, at mile 13.8 of your loop hike. Turn right and begin climbing through second-growth forest dominated by tulip trees. Cross Rough Creek at mile 14.3, then turn well away from the watercourse. Descend to cross the stream again at mile 15.1, then cross a third time. Get water here, at the last source you'll encounter for several miles.

Ascend the slope of Sugarland Mountain, passing through hemlock coves. Rock work on the downside of the trail keeps the path level. Reach Sugarland Mountain Trail at mile 16.6. Turn right here and keep climbing on a knife-edge ridge. The trail eventually decides to stay primarily on the west side of the ridge, affording views into Tennessee.

You'll pass by occasional rock outcrops then, at 17.1 miles, the trail straddles a piney ridge. There are great views to the right of Sweet Ridge, Miry Ridge, and Blanket Mountain in the distance. Red spruce trees begin to appear, indicating high country. You are now at 5,000 feet. Yellow birch with widespread crowns complement the stately spruce trees. Climb to meet Sweet Ridge, and keep pushing, passing the Mount Collins trail shelter spring at mile 20.8. You'll soon reach an intersection with the side trail to the shelter. Sugarland Mountain Trail levels off, then makes a little climb in spruce–fir woods to meet the Appalachian Trail at mile 21.4. Turn right on the A.T. to make a brief climb over Mount Collins before descending to Collins Gap at 22.6 miles. Climb away from Collins Gap and wind your way up to Clingmans Dome. The trailside vegetation is a hodge-podge of brush, grass, and trees. You'll reach the side trail for Clingmans Dome tower at 24.5 miles. Turn left here to reach the observation tower. From there, descend on a paved path to complete your loop at 25 miles.

DIRECTIONS: From Newfound Gap, drive 7 miles to the end of Clingmans Dome Road. Forney Ridge Trail starts at the far end of the Clingmans Dome parking area.

GPS Trailhead Coordinates	34 CLINGMANS DOME OVERNIGHT LOOP
Latitude:	N35° 33' 27.0"
Longitude:	W83° 29' 51.3"
UTM Zone (WGS84):	17S
Easting:	0273640
Northing:	3937560

35 Maddron Bald Overnight Loop

SCENERY: ☆ ☆ ☆ ☆ ☆	DISTANCE (PER DAY): 4.8, 6.2, 6.8 miles
DIFFICULTY: ☆ ☆ ☆	HIKING TIME (PER DAY): 2.75, 3.75, 4 hours
TRAIL CONDITIONS: ☆ ☆ ☆ ☆	OUTSTANDING FEATURES: Henwallow Falls,
SOLITUDE: ☆ ☆ ☆ ☆	old-growth forest, Maddron Bald views
CHILDREN: ☆ ☆	

This two-night trip is one of the best (if not the very best) backpacking loops in the entire park! Hike along the lower reaches of Gabes Mountain, passing Henwallow Falls, and enter virgin woodland to camp at Sugar Cove. Then head up Maddron Bald Trail to Albright Grove, which contains some of the park's largest trees. Camp along a resonant high-country creek near Maddron Bald, which sports awe-inspiring views both above and below. On the return trip down the rugged Snake Den Ridge Trail, a few more vistas open up on some smaller heath balds. This excursion presents the Smoky Mountains at their finest.

Your trip starts on Gabes Mountain Trail. You'll cross several branches of Crying Creek on footlogs before arriving at an old road turnaround at mile 1.1. While climbing the side of Gabes Mountain, pass crumbling homesites scattered in the second-growth woods along the old road. A graded side trail leads to the foot of Henwallow Falls at mile 2.1.

View the falls, then continue right on Gabes Mountain Trail to enter an old-growth forest. Large, slick-surfaced beech trees and huge but imperiled hemlocks stand out among the giants. The trail crosses small brooks that carve through the mountainside and feed the fern and rhododendron understory.

Ford Greenbrier Creek at mile 4.8 and arrive at Sugar Cove Backcountry Campsite 34 (elevation 3,240 feet). This is your first night's destination. The campsite gets a fair amount of use but is in good shape, with camping areas lining the creek.

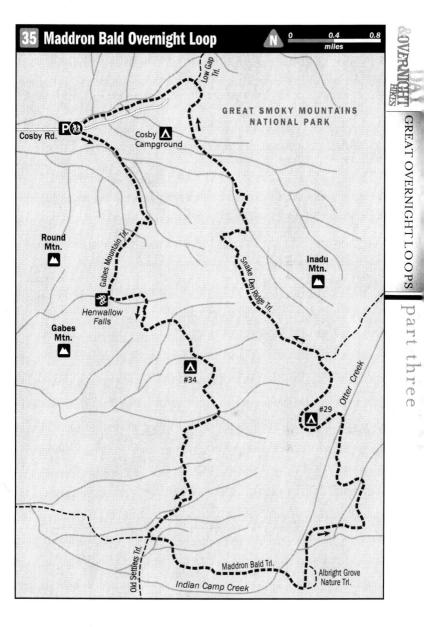

35 Maddron Bald Overnight Loop

N

0   0.4   0.8
miles

GREAT SMOKY MOUNTAINS
NATIONAL PARK

Low Gap Trl.

Cosby Rd.

P

Cosby
Campground

Round
Mtn.

Inadu
Mtn.

Gabes Mountain Trl.

Snake Den Ridge Trl.

Henwallow
Falls

Gabes
Mtn.

#34

#29

Otter Creek

Old Settlers Trl.

Maddron Bald Trl.

Indian Camp Creek

Albright Grove
Nature Trl.

The next day, continue westward on Gabes Mountain Trail. Slowly snake your way along Cole Creek; the trail crosses Cole Creek and its tributaries so many times that you'll think Cole Creek *is* the trail. Don't forget to look up at all the big trees above as you rock-hop over the watercourses. At mile 6.6, the trail arrives at the Maddron Bald Trail junction.

Turn left up Maddron Bald Trail, past the boulder in the middle of the road. Come to an old road turnaround at mile 7.7 of your loop hike. The trail becomes a rocky footpath, crossing Indian Camp Creek on a footlog at mile 8.2. The view up the creek is quite picturesque. Rounding the point of a small ridge, you'll come to Albright Grove Nature Trail at mile 8.3.

Turn right on the nature trail and see some reasons for the establishment of this national park. Old-growth Carolina silverbells, beeches, and tulip trees have been spared the logger's ax and now enjoy national park protection along this 0.7-mile trail, which winds among the giants that lie between Indian Camp and Dunn creeks. Return to Maddron Bald Trail at mile 9.

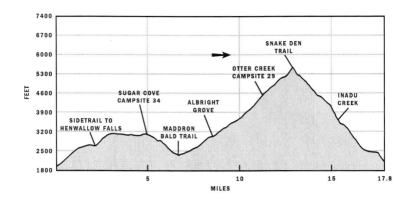

Maddron Bald Trail ascends along, and sometimes through, Indian Camp and Copperhead creeks, leaving the cove to round the point of a ridge at mile 10.5. A small trail to your left emerges at a rocky overlook among crowded brush. From the overlook you can see the town of Cosby below. To your left is Snag Mountain. Up and to your right is Maddron Bald.

Keep ascending on Maddron Bald Trail to reach Otter Creek Backcountry Campsite 29 (elevation 4,560 feet), at mile 11. This is your second night's destination. A small Civilian Conservation Corps camp once occupied this series of small level areas. A pulley-operated food-hanging device, with directions, has been erected for your convenience. The wind rushes through the Otter Creek hollow year-round. Maddron Bald, a mere half mile away, makes a good day hike from the camp.

Day three starts with the climb away from Otter Creek and up to Maddron Bald, at mile 11.5. This heath bald has low, dense bush cover rather than grass cover, but the occasional rock outcrop lets you take in the outstanding views, both near and far. The state-line ridge stands above and to the south; the lower Smokies extend north.

Beyond the bald, reenter the forest and intersect Snake Den Ridge Trail at mile 12.5. This is the high point of the trip (elevation 5,800 feet) as you can tell by the high-country spruce and fir trees. Turn left on Snake Den Ridge Trail and start working your way down a set of switchbacks. Occasionally, on the dry ridgetops, you'll be able to see over the heathlike groundcover to view the crest of the Smokies to your right.

At mile 15.2, the trail crosses Inadu Creek. It then works its way northeast down a cove to cross Rock Creek on a footlog at mile 16.2. Soon the trail comes into an old road turnaround and enters a previously settled area. A trail linking Snake Den Ridge Trail to Low Gap Trail enters from the right at mile 16.8. Turn right and follow the connector trail 0.6 miles to the Low Gap Trail junction.

Turn left and follow Low Gap Trail 0.4 miles down to the hiker parking area at mile 17.8, completing the loop.

DIRECTIONS: From Gatlinburg, take US 321 east to a T-intersection with TN 32. Turn right on TN 32 and follow it a little more than 1 mile, turning right into the signed Cosby section of the park. At 2.1 miles on Cosby Road, arrive at the hiker parking area on the left, near the campground registration hut. Walk back on Cosby Road 0.1 mile to the picnic area to pick up Gabes Mountain Trail across the road.

GPS Trailhead Coordinates	35 MADDRON BALD OVERNIGHT LOOP
Latitude:	N35° 45' 28.0"
Longitude:	W83° 12' 31.0"
UTM Zone (WGS 84):	17S
Easting:	0300310
Northing:	3959130

36 Mount Sterling Overnight Loop

SCENERY: ✿ ✿ ✿ ✿ ✿	DISTANCE (PER DAY): *5.1, 6, 6.2 miles*
DIFFICULTY: ✿ ✿ ✿	HIKING TIME (PER DAY): *3, 4, 3.75 hours*
TRAIL CONDITIONS: ✿ ✿ ✿ ✿	OUTSTANDING FEATURES: *Big Creek, Walnut*
SOLITUDE: ✿ ✿ ✿ ✿	*Bottoms, views from Mount Sterling*
CHILDREN: ✿ ✿ ✿	

Start this trip at Big Creek Ranger Station (an out-of-the-way yet easily accessible departure point) for a trip along Big Creek and into the high country. Follow an old road on a gentle grade to Walnut Bottoms. Camp where several streams come together to provide ample fishing opportunities for those inclined to drop a line. Then climb the rigorous Swallow Fork Trail to the high country on Mount Sterling Ridge. Some pleasant ridge walking leads to Mount Sterling and your second night's destination, at the highest unsheltered backcountry campsite in the park. Pass through old-growth forest on your descent along Baxter Creek Trail and back to Big Creek, where the loop ends.

🏃 To begin, proceed up Big Creek Trail past the gate and follow what was once an Indian footpath, then a logging railroad, and finally an auto road, before it returned to being a horse trail and footpath. Parallel Big Creek, an exceptionally attractive mountain stream, to pass the Rock House on the right at mile 1. Once a home for logging families waiting for better quarters, the Rock House provides welcome shelter from the summer thunderstorms so prevalent in the Smokies.

Mouse Creek Falls spills into Big Creek on your left at mile 2.1. A wide Civilian Conservation Corps bridge spans Big Creek at mile 2.3. One of the Smokies' best-named and most famous springs appears on the left at mile 2.8. Brakeshoe Spring, named for a railroad brake placed there by an engineer with a fondness for Smoky Mountain water, flows on the left. The brake shoe is gone; only the name remains.

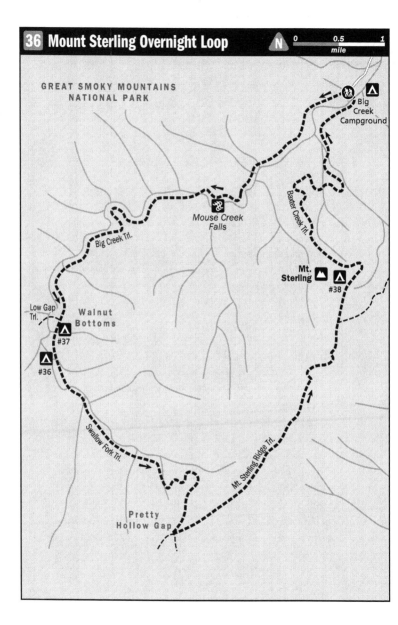

GREAT SMOKY MOUNTAINS
NATIONAL PARK

Big
Creek
Campground

Mouse Creek
Falls

Baxter Creek Trl.

Big Creek Trl.

Mt.
Sterling

#38

Low Gap
Trl.

Walnut
Bottoms

#37

#36

Swallow Fork Trl.

Mt. Sterling Ridge Trl.

Pretty
Hollow Gap

N   0   0.5   1
mile

Continue following Big Creek as it wanders up the valley, and then ford Flint Rock Cove Branch at mile 4.3. At mile 5, come to the Swallow Fork Trail junction. Stay on Big Creek Trail and cross the bridge over Big Creek to enter Lower Walnut Bottoms Backcountry Campsite 37 (elevation 3,000 feet), at mile 5.1, your first night's destination. This campsite is popular with both hikers and bears. Food-storage cables are provided to help keep the bears wild and the hikers in possession of the provisions they brought. Do not leave food lying about!

Begin day two by crossing the bridge back over Big Creek and turning right on Swallow Fork Trail at mile 5.2 of your loop hike. Ascend a gently graded trail to McGinty Creek, where the trail steepens considerably. At mile 6, Swallow Fork Trail crosses Swallow Fork on a footlog. Cross McGinty Creek at mile 6.3; after passing a mountain flat, begin the pull to reach Pretty Hollow Gap. Leave the Swallow Fork hollow and make a sharp right turn at mile 8.5 to switchback up to Pretty Hollow Gap. Here, at mile 9.2, the spruce–fir high country is nearly a mile high.

Turn left on Mount Sterling Ridge Trail, ascending out of

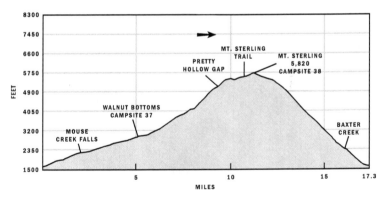

the gap to a small knob flanked by fragrant evergreen trees. Briefly descend, then make the push for Mount Sterling. When you come to the Mount Sterling Trail junction at mile 10.6, pass straight through. The trail changes names at this point, from Mount Sterling Ridge Trail to Mount Sterling Trail. Pass through grassy and forested areas, then beyond a horse-hitch rack on your right, before topping out on Mount Sterling at mile 11.1.

A fire tower tops Mount Sterling, offering a 360-degree view. Be very careful on this (or any other) fire tower. Below the tower is Mount Sterling Backcountry Campsite 38 (elevation 5,800 feet). This is your second night's destination. To get water, descend Baxter Creek Trail, which starts near the fire tower. At about 0.5 miles, look for a spur trail to a spring on the left. Evergreens shelter various designated campsites below the fire tower. Note: The weather can be severe on Mount Sterling any time of the year.

Day three begins with a descent of Baxter Creek Trail through old-growth forest that evokes the Canadian woods. Pass the trail to the spring at mile 11.6 of your loop hike. Switchbacks lead to and beyond the point of Mount Sterling Ridge at mile 13.3. The downgrade remains remarkably consistent until you enter Baxter Creek Valley, where you cross a branch of Baxter Creek at mile 15.6, and then cross Baxter Creek itself at mile 16. Continue along the east bank of Baxter Creek, crossing Big Creek on a footbridge before arriving at the Big Creek picnic area at mile 17.3, completing your loop.

DIRECTIONS: From Interstate 40, take the Waterville Exit 451. Cross the Pigeon River, then turn left to follow the Pigeon upstream. Go 2.3 miles after crossing the Pigeon and come to an intersection. Proceed forward through the intersection and soon enter the park. Pass the Big Creek Ranger Station and come to the Big Creek picnic area at mile 3.4. Park here and backtrack a short distance to the Big Creek trailhead.

GPS Trailhead Coordinates	36 MOUNT STERLING OVERNIGHT LOOP
Latitude:	N35° 45' 7.3"
Longitude:	W83° 6' 36.6"
UTM Zone (WGS 84):	17S
Easting:	0309150
Northing:	3958290

SCENERY: ☆ ☆ ☆ ☆ ☆	DISTANCE (PER DAY): *1.6, 8.3, 9.2 miles*
DIFFICULTY: ☆ ☆ ☆ ☆	HIKING TIME (PER DAY): *1, 4.75, 5 hours*
TRAIL CONDITIONS: ☆ ☆ ☆ ☆	OUTSTANDING FEATURES: *High-country*
SOLITUDE: ☆ ☆ ☆	*ridges, some views, diverse flora and fauna*
CHILDREN: ☆ ☆	

Leave scenic Cataloochee Valley, seeing an old school and former fields before heading up Pretty Hollow to make your first campsite. The next day, continue up a deeply cut gorge reaching spruce forest at Pretty Hollow Gap. From here, join Mount Sterling Ridge and cruise the high country to camp at Laurel Gap shelter, more than 1 mile high. Your last day is your longest as you follow Balsam Mountain then dip into the lowlands via the lush Palmer Creek Trail.

🚶🚶 Cataloochee Valley is enjoying increased popularity these days because of the reintroduction of the majestic elk that now roam the area. (You may see elk pellets along the path.) Before starting the hike, take a minute to examine Beech Grove School, the white board structure just across Palmer Creek. The children of Cataloochee attended school here until the residents were forced to sell their beloved homesteads when the national park was established.

To begin the loop, leave Cataloochee Road on the wide roadbed of the easy-walking Pretty Hollow Gap Trail. Palmer Creek rushes by to your left. Pass the Turkey George horse camp at 0.2 miles, then go around a pole gate to come along some old fields, known as Indian Flats, so named because they were there when the pioneers first set foot in this watershed. It is believed that the native people kept fields such as this open by burning them in order to attract game animals, which they would then slay and eat.

Pass Little Cataloochee Trail at 0.7 miles. Here, Pretty Hollow Creek Trail veers left, passing rock walls and other evidence of

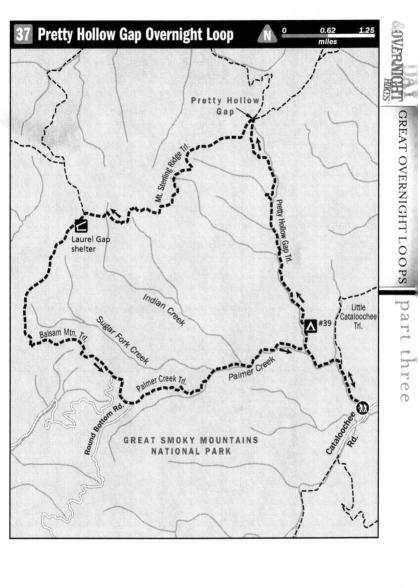

Pretty Hollow
Gap

Mt. Sterling Ridge Trl.

Pretty Hollow Gap Trl.

Laurel Gap
shelter

Indian Creek

Little
Cataloochee
Trl.

#39

Balsam Mtn. Trl.

Sugar Fork Creek

Palmer Creek Trl.

Palmer Creek

Round Bottom Rd.

Cataloochee Rd.

GREAT SMOKY MOUNTAINS
NATIONAL PARK

settlement before intersecting Palmer Creek Trail, your return route, at 1.6 miles. Continue straight, beginning your journey into Pretty Hollow. The ascent is minimal, and soon the path reaches Pretty Hollow Backcountry Campsite 39. This is your first night's destination. The sloped camping area has four designated sites. Imperiled hemlocks grow under pine overstory here, and the uppermost campsite is in oak woods. A horse-hitching rack is just uptrail of the campsite.

The next day you'll ascend from the camp to reach Pretty Hollow Creek and cross it by footlog at 3.1 miles, 3.4 miles, and 3.8 miles of your loop hike. Pass through an imperiled mature hemlock grove, crossing Onion Bed Branch at 4.1 miles. The canopied forest gives way to gorgeous open woodland of beech, buckeye, yellow birch, spruce, and fir, with a grassy carpet for a floor. You'll reach Pretty Hollow Gap, at 5,179 feet, at 5.5 miles. The gap forms a grassy break in Mount Sterling Ridge. Head left on the level Mount Sterling Ridge Trail. Here, Benton MacKaye Trail (BMT) runs in conjunction with the Mount Sterling Ridge Trail. This is a gentle climb amid more grassy woods. The trail soon reaches 5,500 feet and stays at this elevation

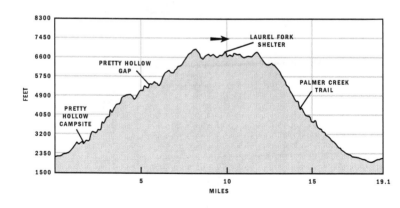

for miles, offering the easiest high-country walking in the park. The slope to your right rises to Big Cataloochee Mountain, at 6,155 feet. Several spring branches flow over the path. The levelness of the trail causes drainage problems in some areas, and the track can be muddy in spots as it wanders through thick stands of red spruce and Fraser fir amid open grassy slopes pocked with wind-stunted birch and maple stands, allowing only occasional views to the south and east. Still other trail sections travel beneath a rhododendron canopy.

You'll reach Balsam Mountain Trail at 9.6 miles. Veer left on Balsam Mountain, walking 0.3 miles to reach the Laurel Gap trail shelter and your second night's destination. A clearing allows you to better appreciate the highland setting. Reservations are required for this shelter, so make sure to call (865) 436-1231 to secure a spot before setting out. Dark-eyed juncos will be flittering about the vicinity in summer. This little gray bird returns to the high country during the spring warm-up then stays in the spruce–fir woods until fall, when it heads to the park's lowlands. This "vertical migration" is its most notable characteristic.

Start day three by continuing on Balsam Mountain Trail, rising past Balsam High Top before descending through grassy forest to meet Beech Gap Trail at 11.3 miles into your loop hike. Stay with Balsam Mountain Trail as it heads more down than up, leaving the spruce–fir high country for deciduous woodlands before meeting gravel Round Bottom Road at Pin Oak Gap at 13.6 miles. Turn left, walking Round Bottom Road to meet Palmer Creek Trail at 14.3 miles. Begin descending the deep forest path on Trail Ridge for a half mile to drop into the steep watershed, crossing Beech Creek on a footlog at 15.9 miles. Palmer Creek's steep slopes prevented the heavy settlement seen in other parts of Cataloochee Valley. The name "Palmer" could've derived from any number of Palmers who settled in Cataloochee Valley, starting with George Palmer in the 1840s. He had many descendants who were also named George, so you could

safely say that the creek was named for "George Palmer" and leave
it at that. At one time, there were so many George Palmers in
Cataloochee that they had to go by nicknames. Stay along the
precipitous mountainside above Palmer Creek, crossing Indian
Creek at 16.3 miles. Continue downhill to reach the bottomland
along Palmer Creek, where red maple, birch, beech, and scads of
rhododendron thrive. Cross Palmer Creek on a footlog before
meeting Pretty Hollow Gap Trail at 17.5 miles. From here, backtrack
1.6 miles to complete your overnight loop.

DIRECTIONS: From Exit 20 on Interstate 40, take NC 276 south
a short distance to Cove Creek Road. Turn right on Cove Creek Road
and follow it nearly 5.7 miles to enter the park. Two miles beyond
the park boundary, turn left onto Cataloochee Road. Follow it
4.1 miles, until it becomes gravel. Pretty Hollow Gap Trail starts
on the right in a parking area just before the gravel road crosses
Palmer Creek.

GPS Trailhead Coordinates	37 PRETTY HOLLOW GAP
	OVERNIGHT LOOP
Latitude:	N35° 37' 36.3"
Longitude:	W83° 6' 47.3"
UTM Zone (WGS 84):	17S
Easting:	0308660
Northing:	3944410

38 Chasteen Creek Overnight Loop

SCENERY: ☆ ☆ ☆ ☆ ☆
DIFFICULTY: ☆ ☆ ☆
TRAIL CONDITIONS: ☆ ☆ ☆ ☆
SOLITUDE: ☆ ☆ ☆
CHILDREN: ☆ ☆

DISTANCE (PER DAY): *3.5, 8.7, 5.2 miles*
HIKING TIME (PER DAY): *2, 4.25, 2.5 hours*
OUTSTANDING FEATURES: *waterfalls, bear country*

This loop travels watercourses and ridges of the Bradley Fork watershed. Leave Smokemont Campground and make your way up Bradley Fork, then turn up Chasteen Creek, where a waterfall awaits along a side trail. Continue to the upper reaches of the stream and overnight at Upper Chasteen Creek Backcountry Campsite. The next day, climb through mountainside woodlands to reach Hughes Ridge. Here, rhododendron and altitude-loving Fraser fir trees line the trail. Take a pleasant stroll in the high country before dropping down Taywa Creek and returning to Bradley Fork. Head up Bradley Fork to camp at Cabin Flats, one of the Smokies' most notorious campsites for frequent bear encounters. Worry not: bear-proof food storage cables have been installed here, as at all other Smokies campsites. Bradley Fork is simply beautiful here and is great for wading, fishing, or simply peering into the crystalline waters. Also, in June, backpackers can achieve a big-bloom "triple crown": flame azalea, mountain laurel, and rhododendron flower along the trails.

🚶🚶 To begin, leave Smokemont Campground. Bradley Fork flows, dashes, and splashes along Bradley Fork Trail, where mossy boulders and ferns lie beneath the forest, with many locust and tulip trees taking over former clearings. Try to imagine the homesites that once occupied these flats. Cross a wooden bridge over Chasteen Creek at mile 1. Just beyond this crossing is the Chasteen Creek Trail junction. Above this small clearing is Lower Chasteen Creek Backcountry Campsite 50.

As you turn right onto Chasteen Creek Trail, the trailbed narrows. Bridge Chasteen Creek again at mile 1.4. The gradient

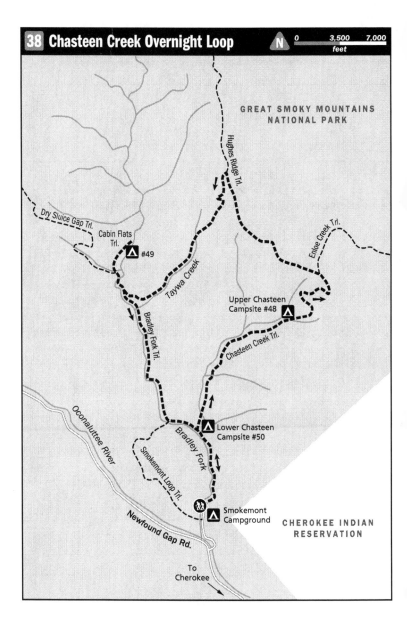

N

0   3,500   7,000
feet

GREAT SMOKY MOUNTAINS
NATIONAL PARK

Hughes Ridge Trl.

Dry Sluice Gap Trl.

Enloe Creek Trl.

Cabin Flats Trl. ▲ #49

Taywa Creek

Upper Chasteen Campsite #48 ▲

Bradley Fork Trl.

Chasteen Creek Trl.

Oconaluftee River

Lower Chasteen Campsite #50 ▲

Bradley Fork

Smokemont Loop Trl.

Smokemont Campground ▲

Newfound Gap Rd.

CHEROKEE INDIAN RESERVATION

To Cherokee

steepens beneath the forest, which has an occasional grassy understory. Other areas are thick with rhododendron. The trail splits near a hitching post at mile 2. A side path leads to Chasteen Creek and a 20-foot cascade tumbling over rocks. Now the path drifts away from the creek, crossing a major feeder branch. Watch for a low-flow cascade emanating from another side stream and passing under the trail. Reach the campsite at mile 3.5 after a short climb. This tiered sloping site—more slope than tier—stands at 3,300 feet. Small streams seemingly encircle the camp.

Start day two by continuing up Chasteen Creek Trail, which steepens and narrows to a single-track footpath. The white noise of falling streams noticeably subsides as you achieve a drier ridgeline, where flame azaleas bloom in June. Small seeps up here may be dry during later summer and fall—water up before you leave the campsite. The path switchbacks among mountain laurel and offers glimpses to the south and west. Reach Hughes Ridge Trail at mile 5 of your loop hike. Turn left here and begin heading mostly uphill in attractive mixed woodland that includes red spruce. Intersect Enloe Creek Trail at mile 5.4 and ascend away from the gap to reach

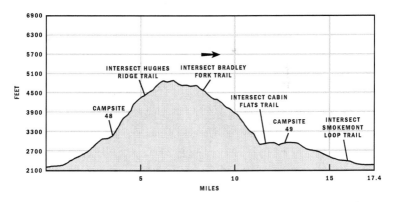

a high point at mile 6.1—you are now at nearly 5,100 feet. Descend through a dark spruce copse, enjoying the path's moderate incline. The high-country ramble continues to head for an attractive junction at mile 7.9, where grass grows amid the trees. Turn left here, descending on the upper portion of Bradley Fork Trail around the point of a ridge, at times tunneling through rhododendron. Bridge Taywa Creek the first time at mile 9.8, and keep steadily descending. Taywa Creek is considered a brook trout stronghold and was formerly off limits to fishing above the trailside waterfall, which acts as a barrier to rainbow trout.

The path turns away from Taywa Creek before reaching a trail junction and a resting bench at mile 11.1. Bradley Fork is crashing on the far side of the rhododendron. Here, pick up Cabin Flats Trail and immediately cross Bradley Fork on an impressive trestle bridge that you will appreciate if the water is high. Cross Tennessee Branch on a footbridge, just beyond which lies the Dry Sluice Gap Trail junction at mile 11.5.

Cabin Flats Trail winds along the west side of Bradley Fork Valley before descending into Cabin Flats proper at mile 12.2, after a sharp right turn. This is the location of Cabin Flats Backcountry Campsite 49. Over the years, this campsite has been closed for periods due to bear activity. Whether bear or human, I would come here to enjoy the beauty of the stream and woods. However, the flood of spring 2003 blew the creekside wide open, and much rock is still exposed. As old as these mountains are, they just keep changing.

Start day three of your loop hike by backtracking 1.1 miles on Cabin Flats Trail to reach Bradley Fork Trail. Keep descending along Bradley Fork, appreciating more of this superlative watercourse on an easy, descending grade. There is an intersection with Smokemont Loop Trail at mile 15.8 of your loop hike. You'll soon reach an intersection with Chasteen Creek Trail then will retrace your steps the last mile of the hike to reach Smokemont and the end of the trail at mile 17.4.

DIRECTIONS: From Oconaluftee Visitor Center, drive 3.2 miles north on Newfound Gap Road to Smokemont Campground. Turn right into the campground on a bridge over the Oconaluftee River. Veer left to pass the campground check-in station. Bradley Fork Trail starts at the gated jeep road at the right rear of the campground.

GPS Trailhead Coordinates	38 CHASTEEN CREEK OVERNIGHT LOOP
Latitude:	N35° 33' 43.2"
Longitude:	W83° 18' 42.5"
UTM Zone (WGS 84):	17S
Easting:	0290450
Northing:	3937650

SCENERY: ☆ ☆ ☆ ☆	DISTANCE (PER DAY): 6.3, 7.0, 9.8 miles
DIFFICULTY: ☆ ☆ ☆	HIKING TIME (PER DAY): 4, 4.75, 5.5 hours
TRAIL CONDITIONS: ☆ ☆ ☆ ☆ ☆	OUTSTANDING FEATURES: Points of historical
SOLITUDE: ☆ ☆ ☆	interest, Deep Creek, ridge walking
CHILDREN: ☆ ☆	

On this trip, you'll head up the famed fishing waters of Deep Creek, the origin of many a Smoky Mountain hunting and fishing tale, to camp on a carpet of pine needles at a streamside site beneath a grove of white pines. You will leave the Deep Creek watershed via the steep Martins Gap Trail, then reach and intersection with Sunkota Ridge Trail for some nice ridge walking to a little-used backcountry campsite, 5,000 feet up on Thomas Ridge. Finally, you'll follow the loop south on the ridge, following Thomas Divide Trail back to Deep Creek.

🏃🏃 Begin the hike on Deep Creek Trail, which starts out as a gravel road, passing the Indian Creek Trail junction at mile 0.7. Cross Indian Creek on a bridge and continue up Deep Creek Trail to a road turnaround at mile 2.2, crossing three bridges and passing the Loop Trail junction along the way. Leave the road to follow a graded trail that traverses Bumgardner Branch, and arrive at Bumgardner Branch Backcountry Campsite 60, at mile 2.9. Stay on the east bank of Deep Creek, which rises far above the creek itself. A historic wagon road once intersected the creek here.

Drop down to McCracken Branch Backcountry Campsite 59, at mile 4.2. Repeat the pattern of rise and fall to enter Nicks Nest Branch Backcountry Campsite 58, at mile 5.7. Trace the right bank of Deep Creek, reaching the historic Bryson Place and a trail junction at mile 6. Once the site of a backwoods cabin and a hunting lodge, this was a favorite haunt of the famed outdoor writer and national park proponent Horace Kephart. Of course,

39 Newton Bald Overnight Loop

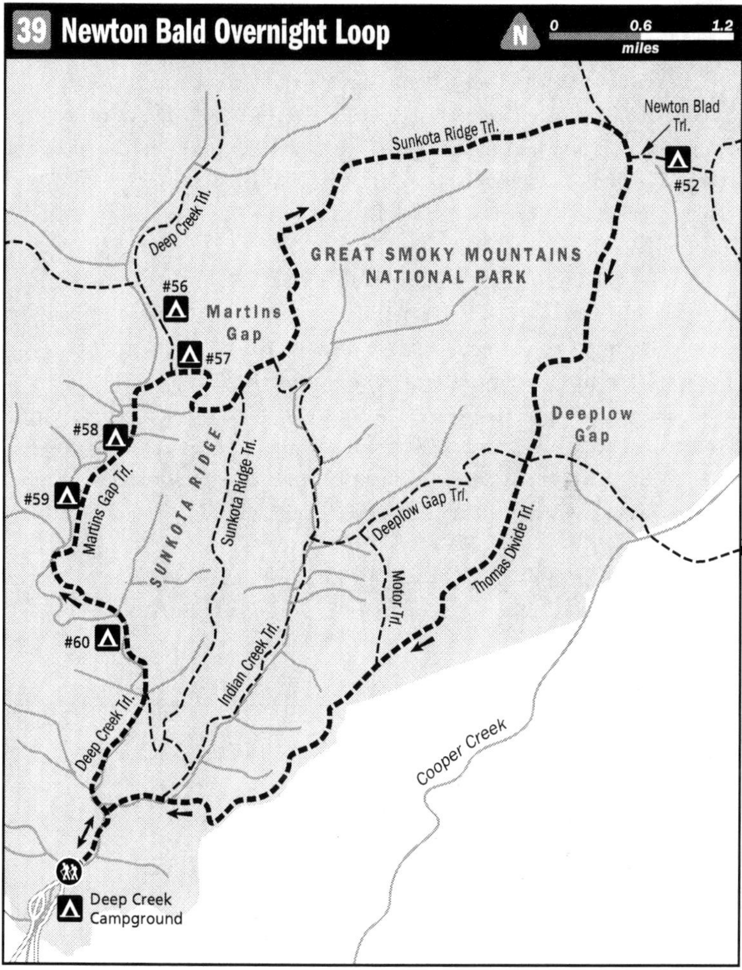
N
0
0.6
1.2
miles
Sunkota Ridge Trl.
Newton Blad Trl.
#52
Deep Creek Trl.
GREAT SMOKY MOUNTAINS NATIONAL PARK
#56
Martins Gap
#57
Deeplow Gap
#58
#59
Martins Gap Trl.
SUNKOTA RIDGE
Sunkota Ridge Trl.
Deeplow Gap Trl.
Motor Trl.
Thomas Divide Trl.
#60
Indian Creek Trl.
Deep Creek Trl.
Cooper Creek
Deep Creek Campground

fishing continues to be a recreational pastime of many Smokies visitors, just as it was in his day.

Leave Bryson Place on Deep Creek Trail and come to Burnt Spruce Backcountry Campsite 56 (elevation 2,405 feet), at mile 6.3. Spend your first night here, under the big white pines, with nearby Deep Creek rushing past. This campsite is nestled between two others that receive heavier usage, Bryson Place and Pole Road; thus it remains a quiet creekside camp.

Day two begins by returning to Bryson Place, 0.3 miles back down Deep Creek Trail. Turn left up Martins Gap Trail, climbing a steep 1.5 miles to its namesake gap at mile 8.1 of your loop hike. Turn left on the infrequently trodden Sunkota Ridge Trail, gently ascending out of Martins Gap around the east side of a knob. Continue ascending, passing a spring at mile 9.5. The trail promises to top out, yet it keeps gaining elevation in moderate spurts between level areas to intersect Thomas Divide Trail at mile 12.9 (elevation 4,780 feet).

Turn right on Thomas Divide Trail and walk 0.4 miles to arrive at Newton Bald Trail junction. Turn left on Newton Bald Trail,

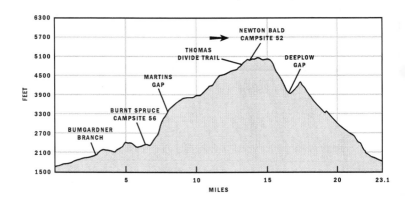

following it 0.1 mile to Newton Bald Backcountry Campsite 52, your second night's destination. This 5,000-foot-high campsite, located in a saddle on Thomas Divide near what was once an open meadow, is a pleasant place to escape the summer heat and crowds. In the winter, Newton Bald is susceptible to strong winds. Chestnut trees still grow on this former bald, but they don't get very big; after a few years, they succumb to the same chestnut blight that essentially wiped out the Smokies' most prolific food-bearing tree species in the 1920s.

Start day three by backtracking 0.1 mile to Thomas Divide Trail. Turn left and begin a southwestward course toward Deep Creek campground. Walk among wooded knolls around 5,000 feet in elevation for nearly 2 miles, then begin a prolonged descent, passing Deeplow Gap Trail at mile 16.5 of your loop hike. Climb out of Deeplow Gap and begin an undulating course along the ridge.

At mile 18.9, your path will intersect what was once Indian Creek Motor Nature Trail; construction began in the 1960s but was halted after a public outcry. The roadbed, running parallel to the park boundary, makes for easy walking as you continually lose elevation. Still on Thomas Divide Trail, you'll come to a trail junction at mile 21. Turn right on Stone Pile Gap Trail and continue your descent, zigzagging over the small creek that often muddies the trail.

Your path intersects the Indian Creek Trail at mile 22; turn left. Pass by Indian Creek Falls on your right, then you'll come to another trail junction at mile 22.4. Turn left on Deep Creek Trail and follow it 0.7 miles to complete your 23.1-mile loop.

DIRECTIONS: From Oconaluftee Visitor Center, take US 441 south to Cherokee, North Carolina. Turn right on US 19 and drive 10 miles to Bryson City, North Carolina. Turn right at the Swain County Courthouse onto Everett Street and carefully follow the signs through town to Deep Creek Campground. Deep Creek Trail starts on the left bank of the stream, across from the campground and beyond the picnic area.

GPS Trailhead Coordinates	39 NEWTON BALD OVERNIGHT LOOP
Latitude:	N35° 27' 34.6"
Longitude:	W83° 26' 18.6"
UTM Zone (WGS 84):	17S
Easting:	0278722
Northing:	3926527

40 Forney Creek Overnight Loop

SCENERY: ✿ ✿ ✿ ✿ ✿	DISTANCE (PER DAY): 9.9, 5.9 or 6.3, 3.2 or 3.6 miles
DIFFICULTY: ✿ ✿ ✿ ✿	HIKING TIME (PER DAY): 6, 3.75, 2 hours
TRAIL CONDITIONS: ✿ ✿ ✿	OUTSTANDING FEATURES: Vistas from
SOLITUDE: ✿ ✿ ✿	Andrews Bald, sites of interest in logging and pioneer
CHILDREN: ✿	history, varied ecosystems

This is a tough but rewarding trek, involving numerous creek fords and an elevation change of more than 4,000 feet! Strap your shoes on for this hike because you have a long first day. Leave Clingmans Dome and travel Forney Ridge, passing Andrews Bald, with its wonderful views. Continue down Forney Ridge to make Civilian Conservation Corps (CCC) Campsite 71 on Forney Creek. The campsite is has a limited number of reservable sites, so call (865) 436-1231 to reserve a spot. Turn up Forney Creek, ascending a great valley along a scintillating mountain stream. Forney Creek has several fords, which can be challenging when the water is high. You have two choices for your second night's destination—Steeltrap—camping either in a seldom-used clearing or beside Forney Creek Cascades. Your final day sees you climb back into the spruce–fir high country that cloaks only the highest elevations of the Smokies.

🚶🚶 To begin this hike, you'll leave Clingmans Dome parking area on Forney Ridge Trail, which is bordered by big boulders, Fraser fir, and mountain ash. Bear left after meeting Clingmans Dome Bypass Trail. The rough, rocky track winds in and out of shade. Open areas allow views. Spruce and fir grow in dense thickets elsewhere, along with yellow birch. Meet Forney Creek Trail, your return route, at 1.2 miles. At 1.8 miles, open onto the upper end of Andrews Bald. Blueberries, azaleas, and rhododendron bushes dot the grassy area, where you can look south to Fontana Lake and waves of mountains beyond. Spur trails lead to other vista spots. Stay right on Forney Ridge Trail, heading down the partially open bald and

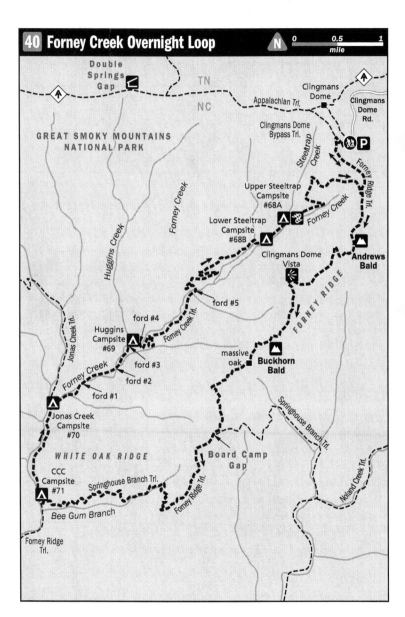

N

0   0.5   1
mile

Double
Springs
Gap

TN

Clingmans
Dome

Clingmans
Dome
Rd.

Appalachian Trl.

NC

GREAT SMOKY MOUNTAINS
NATIONAL PARK

Clingmans Dome
Bypass Trl.

Steeltrap Creek

Forney Ridge Trl.

Upper Steeltrap
Campsite
#68A

Forney Creek

Forney Creek

Lower Steeltrap
Campsite
#68B

Clingmans Dome
Vista

Andrews
Bald

FORNEY RIDGE

Huggins Creek

ford #5

ford #4

Jonas Creek Trl.

Huggins
Campsite
#69

Forney Creek Trl.

massive
oak

Buckhorn
Bald

ford #3

ford #2

Forney Creek

ford #1

Springhouse Branch Trl.

Jonas Creek
Campsite
#70

Noland Creek Trl.

WHITE OAK RIDGE

Board Camp
Gap

CCC
Campsite
#71

Springhouse Branch Trl.

Forney Ridge Trl.

Bee Gum Branch

Forney Ridge
Trl.

gaining views of Welch Ridge and Forney Ridge. Beyond the bald, the trail, shrouded by trees and brush, receives much less use. Work your way downhill, making a hard switchback to the left before rejoining the ridgetop, still more than a mile high. There is not always a tree canopy overhead, so brambles and briars will grow in summer. Occasional spinelike rock protrusions emerge from the trailside.

At 3.1 miles, as you curve around a knob, a view of Clingmans Dome opens to the right. Keep descending, leaving the spruce trees of the high country to head into oak woods. The trail runs along the crest of or else to the right of Forney Ridge, heading continually downhill amid occasional pockets of rhododendron. Here, like everywhere else in the Smokies, the hemlocks are dying.

In a level gap, at 4.5 miles, the trail passes a massive oak tree. From here, Forney Ridge Trail gently undulates, passing beneath now-wooded Buckhorn Bald. You'll reach Board Camp Gap and join Springhouse Branch Trail at 5.8 miles. The junction is a nice place for a break, with a level area and trees to lean against. From Board Camp Gap, the trail undulates on a narrow wooded ridge then makes a hard switchback right at 7.1 miles, leaving Forney Ridge.

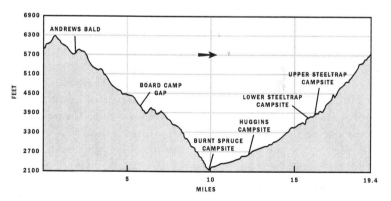

Wind in and out of hollows, crossing the headwaters of Bee Gum Branch at 7.7 miles. Hike west in this valley, staying well above Bee Gum Branch, alternately entering moist hollows and drier mountain laurel, oak, and sassafras woods.

You keep hearing water, and think you're almost there. After a last couple of switchbacks, you'll reach the CCC campsite, elevation 2,160 feet, at 9.9 miles. You will see a large chimney and metal artifacts at this former homesite and CCC camp. The CCC workers who built the trail you just walked were headquartered here. This camp, open to hikers and equestrians, is your first night's destination. Forney Creek rumbles nearby, providing a place to fish or swim. Follow the railroad grade upstream to an old stone trestle at the creek's edge to find two large pools.

Start day two by turning up Forney Creek Trail as it veers away from the stream; this way you'll avoid fords. Next, the trail descends toward a former logging railroad grade, at 10.7 miles into the loop hike. The trail becomes quite rocky before intersecting Jonas Creek Trail at 11.1 miles. Jonas Creek Campsite is just on the other side of the bridge from Forney Creek Trail. Forney Creek Trail is closed to horses from this point forward. Continue up the lush valley bordered by doghobble, mountain laurel, and rhododendron, passing through huge flats.

Ford Forney Creek at 11.6 miles and 12.1 miles. Continue up the right bank to reach the third ford, and Huggins Campsite 69, at 12.4 miles. This backcountry campsite was previously known as Monteith Camp. After the fourth ford, just beyond Huggins, the trailbed becomes wet and rocky. Make a switchback past an enormous rock retaining wall that remains from the railroad days. The trail is well above the stream after you make another switchback. Reach the fifth ford at 14 miles. This crossing takes you to the left-hand bank. More switchbacks lie ahead, entering the great cove hardwood forests where tulip trees grow straight and tall. This railroad grade was made gentle enough for tree-loaded flatcars to ascend the mountains;

therefore, a backpacker loaded with camping gear should be able to make it as well.

You'll reach Lower Steeltrap Campsite 68B at 15.9 miles, not long after you cross Steeltrap Creek. A clearing has a single fire ring, and Steeltrap Creek flows loudly off to your right. Upper Steeltrap Campsite sits at 4,250 feet; Campsite 68A is up the trail 0.4 miles at 16.3 miles, near Forney Creek Cascades. This site has old railroad artifacts, including wheels and rail. The cascades are a wide rockslide about 50 to 60 feet high, with another fall above it. Interestingly, you can see the striations of quartz running through the rock here. Either campsite is your second night's destination.

Start day three by crossing the uppermost section of Forney Creek one last time; it's an easy step over. You'll continue to encounter railroad artifacts here. Portions of the rocky trailside become grassy, and a northern hardwood forest of beech, sugar maple, and yellow birch mixes with spruce and occasional fir trees. Follow the curving path into a watery rock garden to make a big switchback away from the water. Next, climb a wet rocky track, making a last hard switchback to the right before reaching Forney Ridge Trail at 18.3 miles. From here, backtrack 1.2 miles to Clingmans Dome, completing your overnight loop.

DIRECTIONS: From Newfound Gap, drive 7 miles to the end of Clingmans Dome Road. Forney Ridge Trail starts at the tip end of the Clingmans Dome parking area.

GPS Trailhead Coordinates	40 FORNEY CREEK OVERNIGHT LOOP
Latitude:	N35° 33' 27.0"
Longitude:	W83° 29' 51.3"
UTM Zone (WGS 84):	17S
Easting:	0273640
Northing:	3937560

41 Fontana Overnight Loop

SCENERY: ✿ ✿ ✿ ✿ ✿	DISTANCE (PER DAY): *4.5, 8.9, 8.1 miles*
DIFFICULTY: ✿ ✿	HIKING TIME (PER DAY): *2.75, 5, 4.25 hours*
TRAIL CONDITIONS: ✿ ✿ ✿ ✿	OUTSTANDING FEATURES: *Lakeside camping,*
SOLITUDE: ✿ ✿ ✿	*sites of pioneer history; good hike to initiate new*
CHILDREN: ✿ ✿ ✿	*backpackers*

If you like a combination of mountains and lakes, this moderate hike is for you and any younger or inexperienced backpackers you may wish to bring along—though the mileages may be a bit challenging for the uninitiated. Start your trip on a boat that takes you on the pleasure ride from Fontana Marina to Hazel Creek. Hike up a modest grade on Hazel Creek Trail through a valley steeped in settler and logging history to camp at Sugar Fork, one of the Smokies' best campsites. Then backtrack down Hazel Creek to cross over into the Eagle Creek watershed on a newer section of Lakeshore Trail to camp on Fontana Lake and simultaneously enjoy a tumbling stream and a mountain-rimmed lake. On the way back, pass more human history, still on Lakeshore Trail, to reach the intersection with the Appalachian Trail, then walk over Fontana Dam, the highest in the East, to Fontana Marina.

🏃 Before you leave, contact Fontana Marina at (828) 498-2211, extension 277, to arrange for a one-way shuttle; you will hike back to the marina. Start your trip at the mouth of Hazel Creek on Hazel Creek Trail. Pass Proctor Creek Backcountry Campsite 86, at mile 0.5. You'll soon cross Hazel Creek on a wide bridge. The house beside the creek, the Calhoun Place, is owned and used by the park. The newer portion of Lakeshore Trail heads west past the house. Remember this spot, as you will be backtracking to here. Hike along the jeep road and watch for the many signs of the homestead and logging days.

As you hike, the scenic mountain stream is often visible and makes itself heard even when it cannot be seen. Cross two wide bridges before arriving at Sawdust Pile Backcountry Campsite 85,

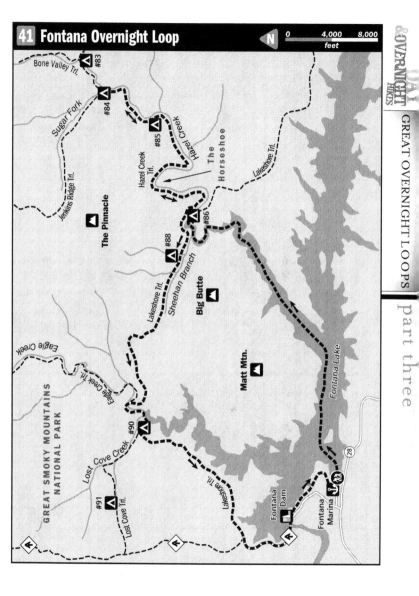

41 Fontana Overnight Loop

N

0   4,000   8,000
feet

Bone Valley Trl.   #83

Sugar Fork

#84

#85

Hazel Creek

Hazel Creek Trl.

The Horseshoe

Lakeshore Trl.

Jenkins Ridge Trl.

The Pinnacle

#86

#88

Lakeshore Trl.

Sheehan Branch

Big Butte

Matt Mtn.

Fontana Lake

Eagle Creek

Eagle Creek Trl.

Lost Cove Creek

#90

GREAT SMOKY MOUNTAINS NATIONAL PARK

#91   Lost Cove Trl.

Lakeshore Trl.

Fontana Dam

Fontana Marina

28

on your right at mile 3.3. Span two more bridges before coming to a trail junction at mile 4.5. To your right, just across the bridge over Sugar Fork, is Sugar Fork Backcountry Campsite 84, at an elevation of 2,160 feet. This is your first night's destination. Nestled between Sugar Fork and Hazel Creeks, this level campsite beneath the pines makes an ideal base camp for the angler or amateur archaeologist. Consider walking up to Bone Valley or up Sugar Fork on Jenkins Ridge Trail, exploring Hazel Creek Valley's past. But leave anything you find.

Start day two by backtracking downstream along Hazel Creek, appreciating the many cascades of this stream that exemplify the beauty of this national park. At mile 8.4 of your loop hike, stay on the west side of Hazel Creek on Lakeshore Trail as it passes by the Calhoun Place. Climb along a bluff then descend again. Remnants of the old community of Proctor, including chimneys, walls, and foundations, are very evident along the valley of Sheehan Branch. You can visit Proctor Cemetery via a side trail at mile 8.9 and pass the newer backcountry campsite 88 on a spur trail leading off Lakeshore Trail. The lower part of this valley was known as Possum Hollow.

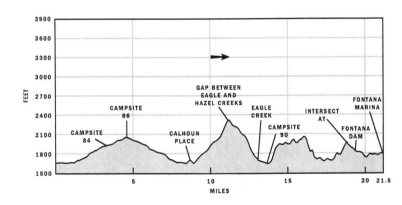

Continue up an old wagon road along an ever-diminishing watercourse to reach a gap at nearly 2,400 feet at mile 10.9. From here, Lakeshore Trail was graded by park personnel to level the footpath. Descend through hickory—oak and pine woods. Many pines are dead from Southern pine beetle infestations in the early 21st century. Watch for boulders on the ridgeline as you traverse small gaps. Briefly travel along a streamlet to emerge along Eagle Creek at mile 12.8. The rushing sounds contrast with the quiet woods of the ridgetop. Turn left to descend along Eagle Creek and cross a metal-frame bridge. Veer right, and the lake comes into view on your left. Pass over Lost Cove Creek on a footlog to arrive at Lost Cove Backcountry Campsite 90 (elevation 1,760 feet) at mile 13.4. This is your second night's destination. This popular campsite extends out beyond the trees and offers fishing and swimming in both Fontana Lake and mountain streams nearby.

Start day three by finding Lost Cove Trail. As you look out on the lake from the campsite, Lost Cove Trail will be uphill and to your right. Follow the trail 0.4 miles to Lakeshore Trail junction. Turn left on Lakeshore Trail. This portion of Lakeshore Trail has many old roads and trails leading off it, so make sure you stay on the right path. Fontana Lake will be on your left the whole way.

The trail follows a familiar pattern: up and around a point of a ridge, and down into a creek-filled hollow; up the side of a ridge and over the point, and down again into a hollow. At mile 16.7 of your loop hike, intersect a former road, Old NC 28. It still has some junker cars from the 1930s nearby. Homesites and other evidence of human habitation are all around this section of trail. Leave the old road at mile 18.5, and climb to another old road that leads to Fontana Dam Road at mile 19.2. The road will intersect the Appalachian Trail at Lakeshore Trail parking area.

Walk along the road to reach the north side of Fontana Dam at mile 19.7. Cross Fontana Dam, appreciating the immensity of the project and the views of Fontana Lake. Follow the Appalachian Trail to the left, away from Fontana Dam Road, and reenter woodland. Pass a trail shelter known as the Fontana "Hilton" because it is so fancy. After running a low ridgeline through thick woods, the A.T. crosses a road leading to the marina, which is a short distance downhill to your left. Turn left on the road to complete your loop at mile 21.5.

DIRECTIONS: From Townsend, Tennessee, take US 321 north to Foothills Parkway and follow it to US 129. Turn south on US 129 into North Carolina. Turn left on NC 28, passing Fontana Village. Go 1.5 miles past the Fontana Village entrance and turn left at the sign to Fontana Dam. Next, turn right at the sign to Fontana Village Marina a short distance on. From Bryson City, North Carolina, take US 19 south to NC 28 and follow it nearly 25 miles to turn right at the sign to Fontana Dam, then right again to reach Fontana Village Marina.

GPS Trailhead Coordinates	41 FONTANA OVERNIGHT LOOP
Latitude:	N35° 26' 28.7"
Longitude:	W83° 47' 38.2"
UTM Zone (WGS 84):	17S
Easting:	0246380
Northing:	3925370

Index

Page references followed by *m* indicate a map.

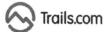
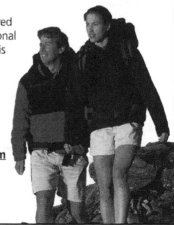

About the Author

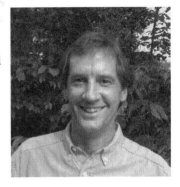

JOHNNY MOLLOY is an outdoor writer based in Johnson City, Tennessee. Born in Memphis, he moved to Knoxville in 1980 to attend the University of Tennessee. During his college years, he developed a love of the natural world that has become the primary focus his life.

It all started on a backpacking foray into Great Smoky Mountains National Park. That first trip was a disaster; nevertheless, Johnny discovered a love of the outdoors that would lead him to canoe-camp and backpack throughout the United States and abroad over the next 25 years. Today, he averages 150 nights out per year.

After graduating from UT in 1987 with a degree in economics, Johnny spent an ever-increasing amount of time in the wild, becoming more skilled in a variety of environments. Friends enjoyed his adventure stories; one even suggested that he write a book. He pursued that idea and soon parlayed his love of the outdoors into an occupation.

The results of his efforts are more than 30 books, including hiking, camping, paddling, and other comprehensive guidebooks, as well as books on true outdoor adventures. He has also written numerous articles for magazines and Web sites, and he continues to write and travel extensively to all four corners of the United States, endeavoring in a variety of outdoor pursuits. For the latest on Johnny, visit his Web site, www.johnnymolloy.com.

AMERICAN HIKING SOCIETY

Because you
hike.
We're with you
every step of the way

American Hiking Society gives voice to the more than 75 million Americans who hike and is the only national organization that promotes and protects foot trails, the natural areas that surround them and the hiking experience. Our work is inspiring and challenging, and is built on three pillars:

Volunteerism and Stewardship: We organize and coordinate nationally recognized programs – including Volunteer Vacations, National Trails Day® and the National Trails Fund –that help keep our trails open, safe and enjoyable.

Policy and Advocacy: We work with Congress and federal agencies to ensure funding for trails, the preservation of natural areas, and the protection of the hiking experience.

Outreach and Education: We expand and support the national constituency of hikers through outreach and education as well as partnerships with other recreation and conservation organizations.

Join us in our efforts. Become an American Hiking Society member today!

American
Hiking
Society

1422 Fenwick Lane · Silver Spring, MD 20910 · (301) 565-6704
www.AmericanHiking.org · info@AmericanHiking.org

DEAR CUSTOMERS

SUPPORTING YOUR INTEREST IN OUTDOOR ADVENTURE, travel, and an active lifestyle is central to our operations, from the authors we choose to the locations we detail to the way we design our books. Menasha Ridge Press was incorporated in 1982 by a group of veteran outdoorsmen and professional outfitters. For 25 years now, we've specialized in creating books that benefit the outdoors enthusiast.

Almost immediately, Menasha Ridge Press earned a reputation for revolutionizing outdoors- and travel-guidebook publishing. For such activities as canoeing, kayaking, hiking, backpacking, and mountain biking, we established new standards of quality that transformed the whole genre, resulting in outdoor-recreation guides of great sophistication and solid content. Menasha Ridge continues to be outdoor publishing's greatest innovator.

The folks at Menasha Ridge Press are as at home on a white-water river or mountain trail as they are editing a manuscript. The books we build for you are the best they can be, because we're responding to your needs. Plus, we use and depend on them ourselves.

We look forward to seeing you on the river or the trail. If you'd like to contact us directly, join in at www.trekalong.com or visit us at www.menasharidge.com. We thank you for your interest in our books and the natural world around us all.

SAFE TRAVELS,

BOB SEHLINGER
PUBLISHER